# The Fate of the Dragon:
## An Illustrated Essay on
## the New Normal

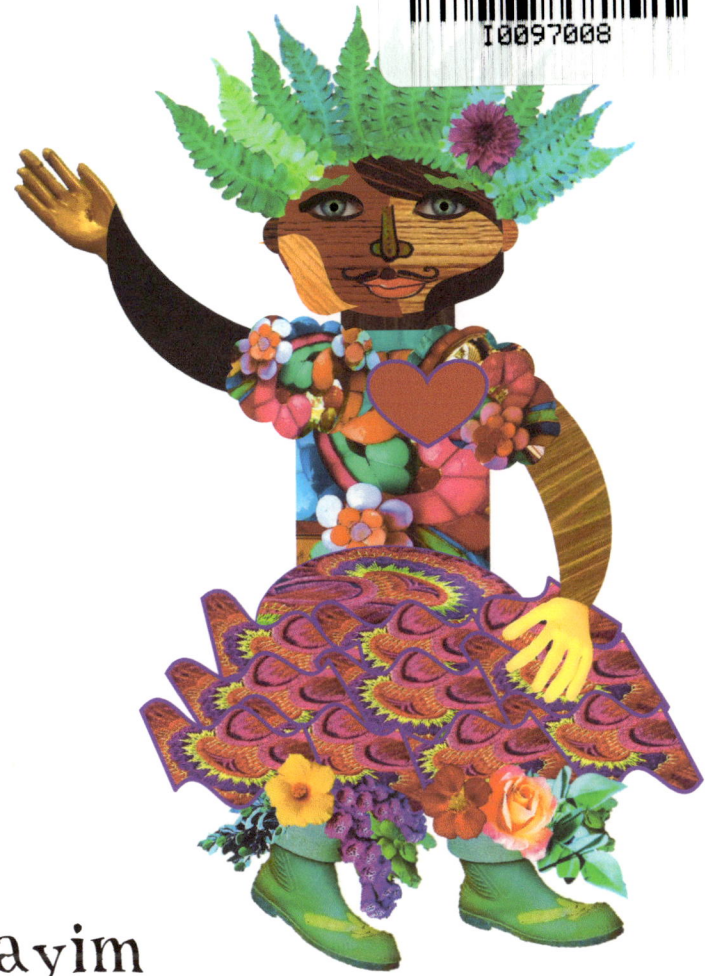

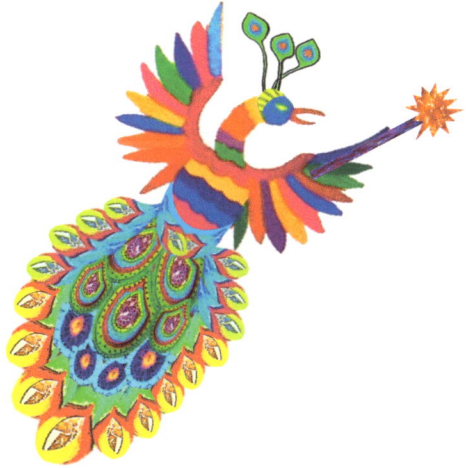

Jordana Chana Mayim

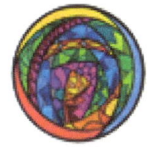

MOSAIC
STREET
PRESS

To get in touch with the publisher, please email us at hello@mosaicstreetpress.com
To get in touch with the author, please email her at jordanamayim@yahoo.com

Book designer: David Adrian Rivero
Proofreader: Rachel Small
Mosaic Street Press logo designer: ÂGrizon

Thank you to those who held on when I wanted to let go.
Thank you to those who support my work.
Thank you to the child who I was, who fought for my right to be who I am. You won.

First Edition

Publisher's Cataloging-in-Publication Data

Names: Mayim, Jordana Chana, author, illustrator.
Title: The fate of the dragon : an illustrated essay on the new normal / Jordana Chana Mayim.
Description: Narberth, PA : Mosaic Street Press, 2022. | Summary: The Fate of the Dragon is an
        illustrated essay on the topic of normality. | Audience: Grades 7 & up.
Identifiers: LCCN 2021917960 (print) | ISBN 978-1-948267-14-4 (paperback) | ISBN 978-1-948267-15-1
        (hardcover) | ISBN 978-1-948267-16-8 (ebook)
Subjects: LCSH: Young adult fiction. | Illustrated works. | CYAC: Suicidal behavior--Fiction. | Mental
        health--Fiction. | Individual differences--Fiction. | Conduct of life--Fiction. | BISAC: YOUNG
        ADULT FICTION / Health & Daily Living / General. | YOUNG ADULT FICTION / Social Themes
        / General.
Classification: LCC PZ7.1.M39 Fat 2022 (print) | LCC PZ7.1.M39 (ebook) | DDC [Fic]--dc23.

To those on the borders
and the precipice of the abyss:

YOU ARE LOVED.
YOU ARE NEEDED.
YOU ARE NOT ALONE.

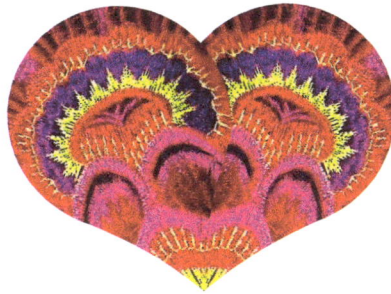

And to MayMariposa:

YOU ARE A MAGICIAN.
And your magic helped transform my life.
GRACIAS Y NAMASTE.

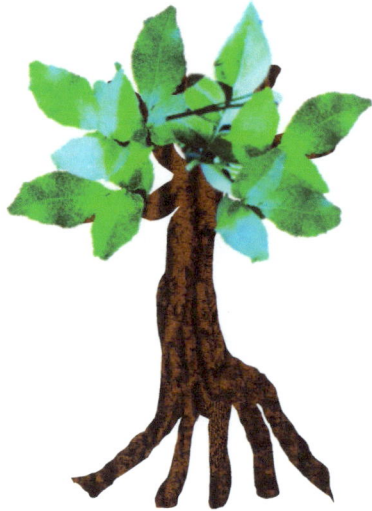

Our fate is in
each other's hands.

UBUNTU:

I am because we are.

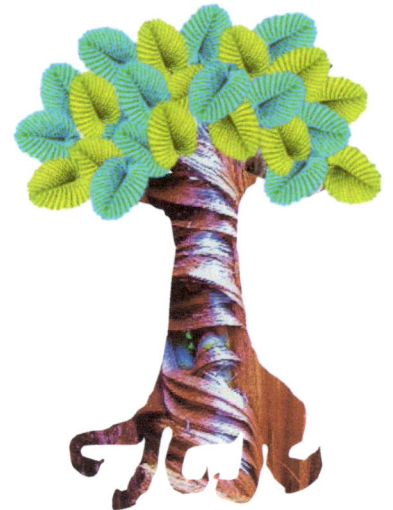

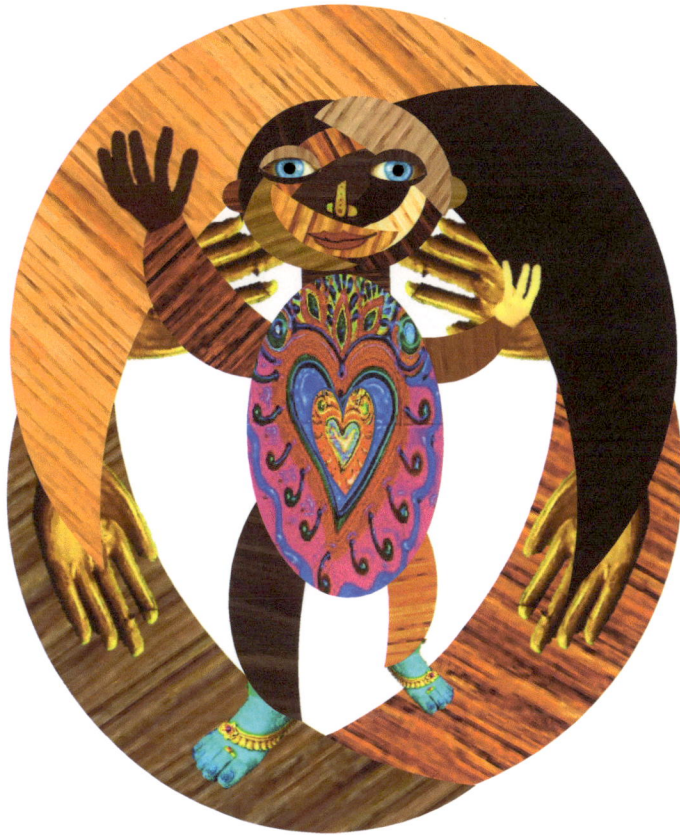

Gaslight:
to manipulate someone
psychologically
so that the person doubts
the legitimacy
of their own
thoughts,
feelings,
memories
and
experiences.

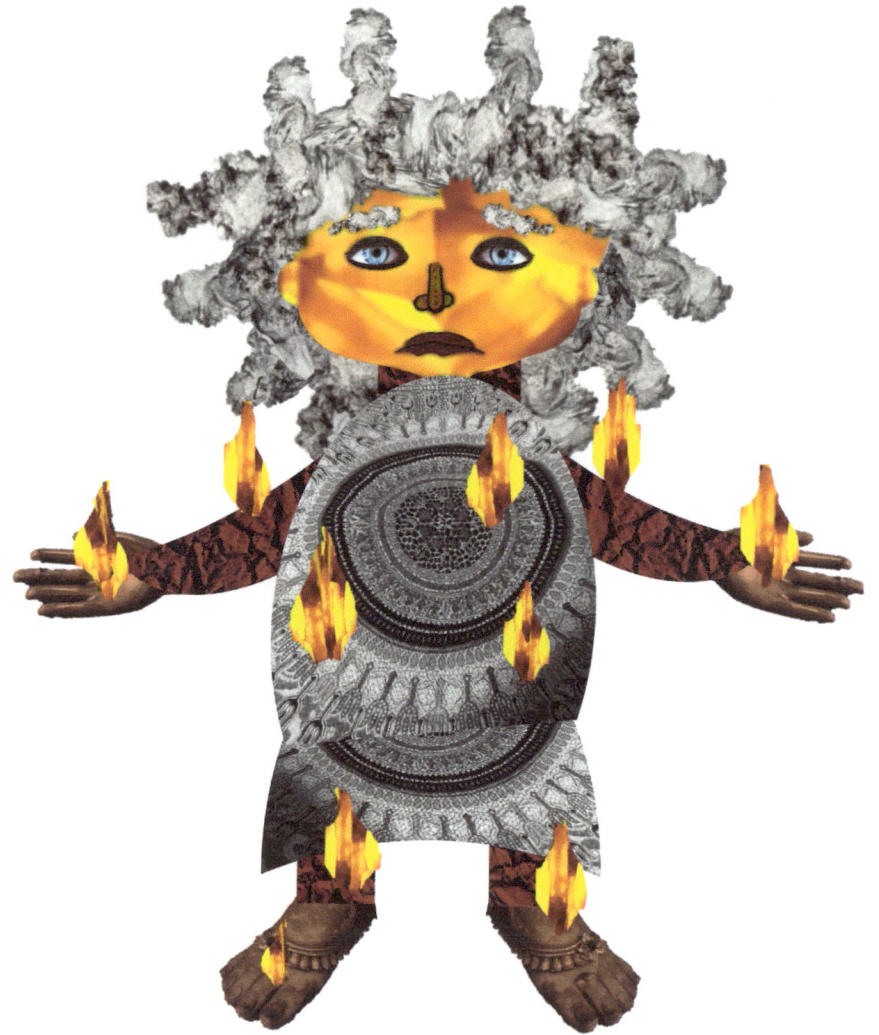

# The Fate of the Dragon

*The* new *normal*.

The words set me seething.
And if I continue to be what I have been,
a prisoner of lies,
I will do with my rage what all the
gaslighted dragons do with their fire:

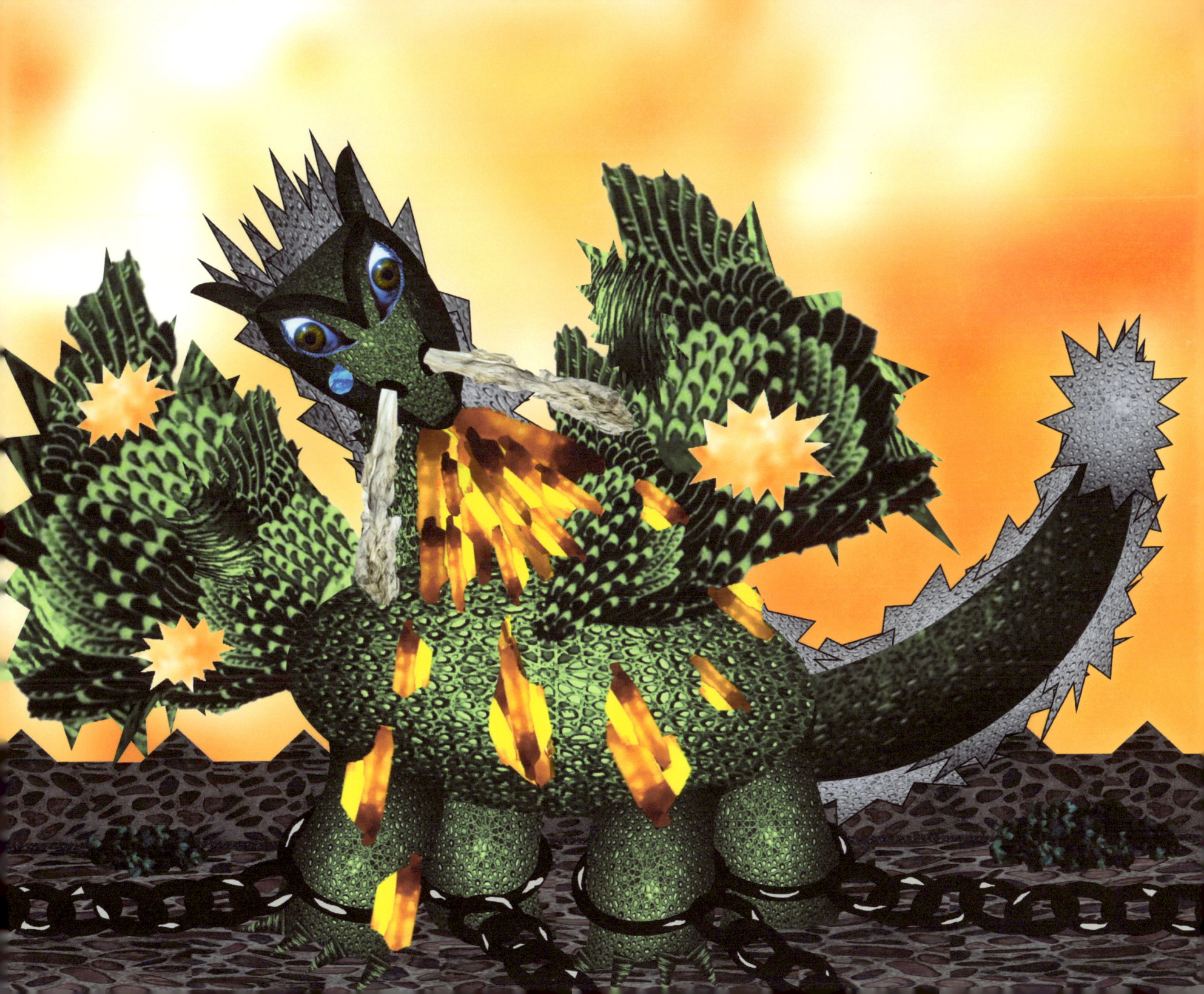

I will incinerate myself.

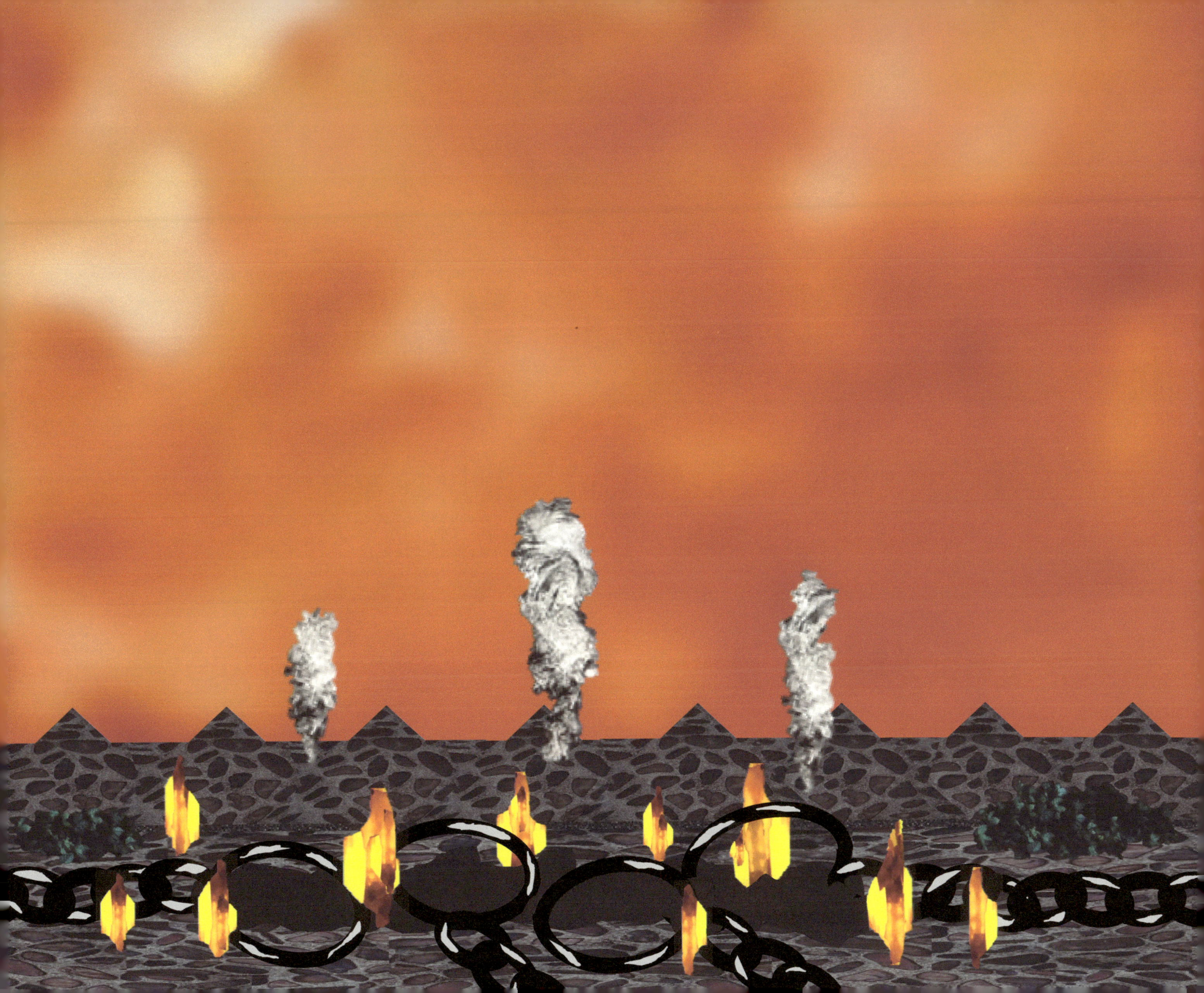

Beside my ashes, discovered in the castle's courtyard,
claw-marked chains will bear proof:
I fought valiantly against vicious foes.

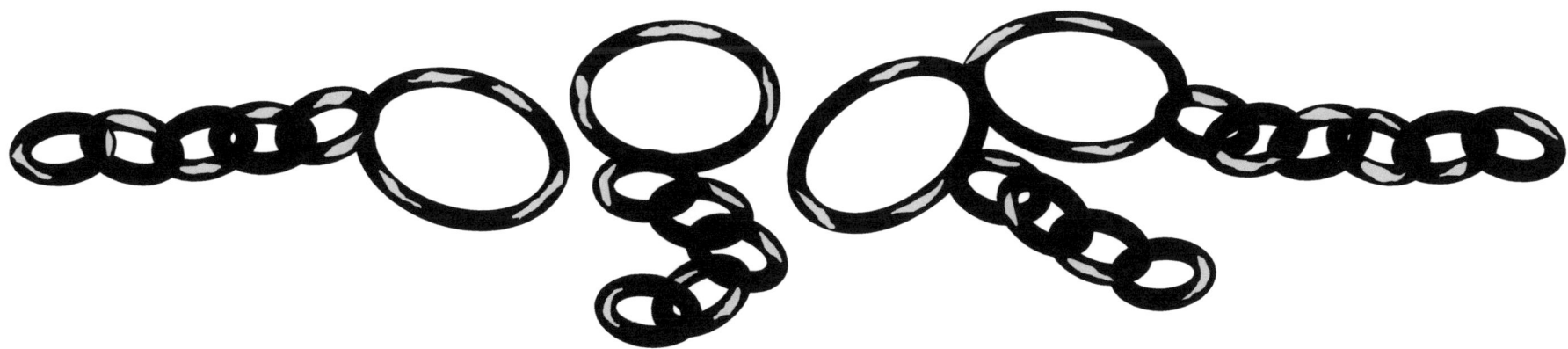

Tear-drenched apologies
and shredded dreams
will precede and follow
my far-too-early exit from this world.

I'm sorry.

I wish
you had told me.

I wish
I had known.

I wish you knew...

Now you'll never...

I wish...

Now we'll never...

I miss you.

I hate you.

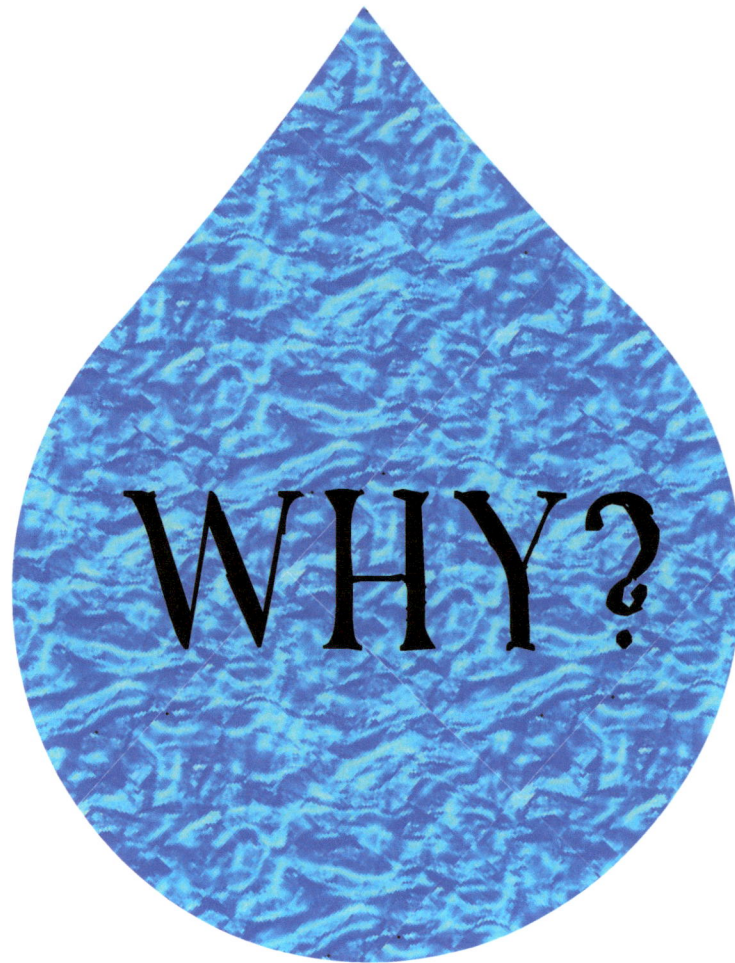

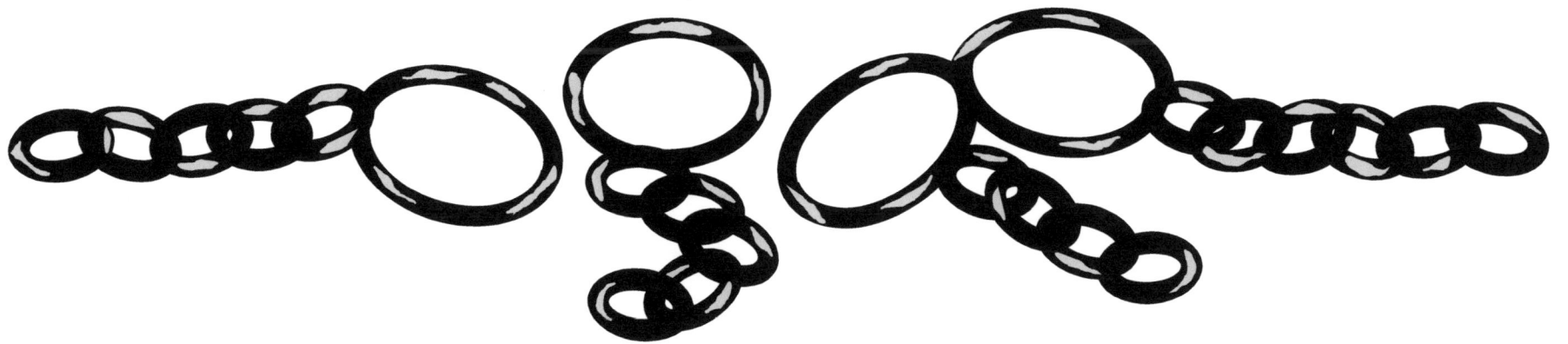

"Forgive me,

but...

No, princess,
I will not rescue you from your tower,
be the wings you need until you repair your own,
be the journey to your crown
and a witness at your coronation
as you dub yourself
*Commander of My Own Steps.*

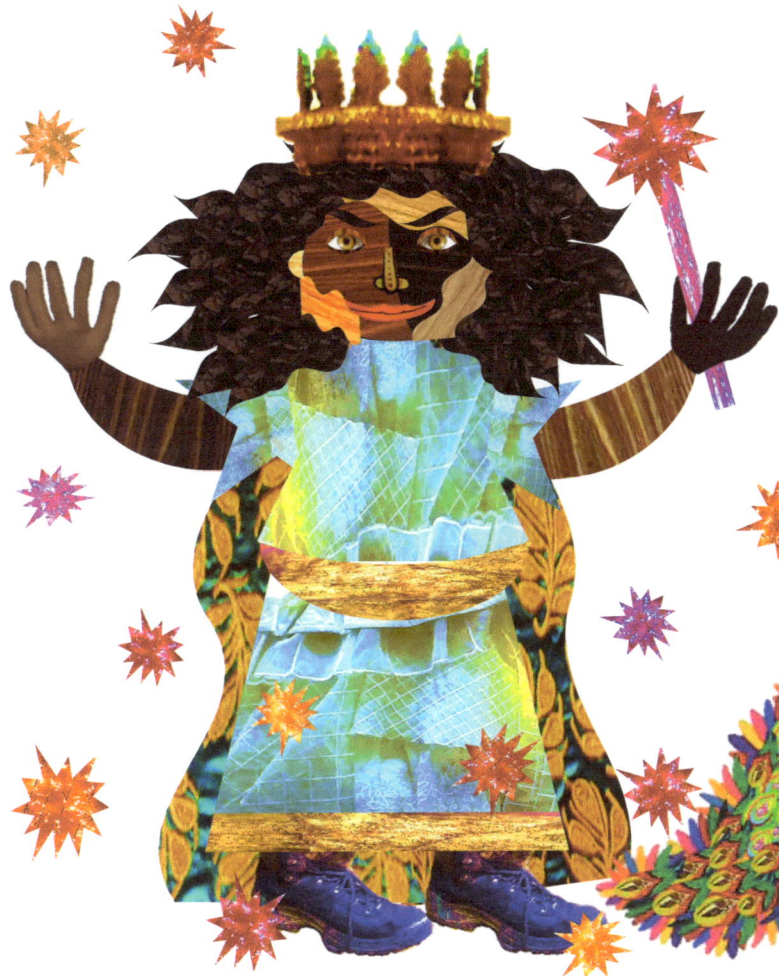

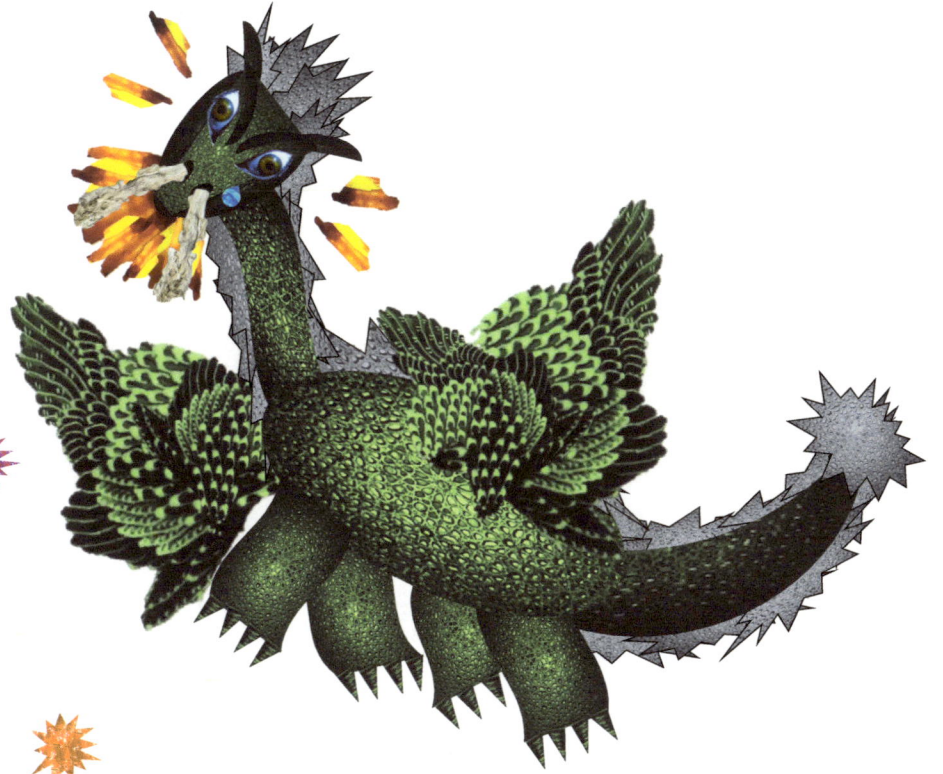

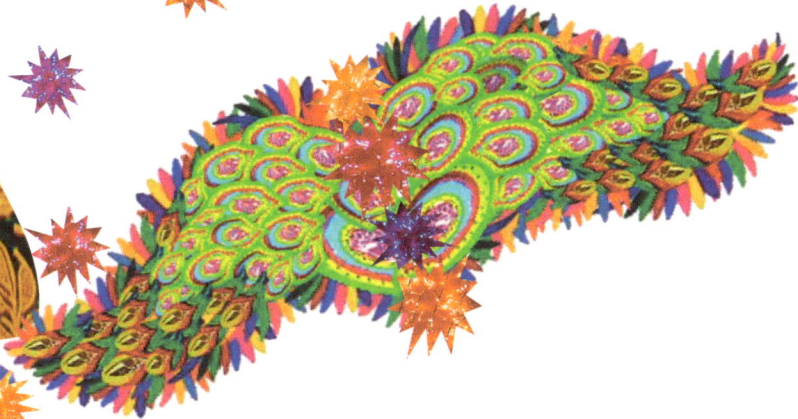

No, subjects,
I will not be your partner in a battle for freedom,
burning up the edicts of a heartless king
and his court of thieves,
ushering justice through the breached fortress walls,
calling upon compassion to author new laws.

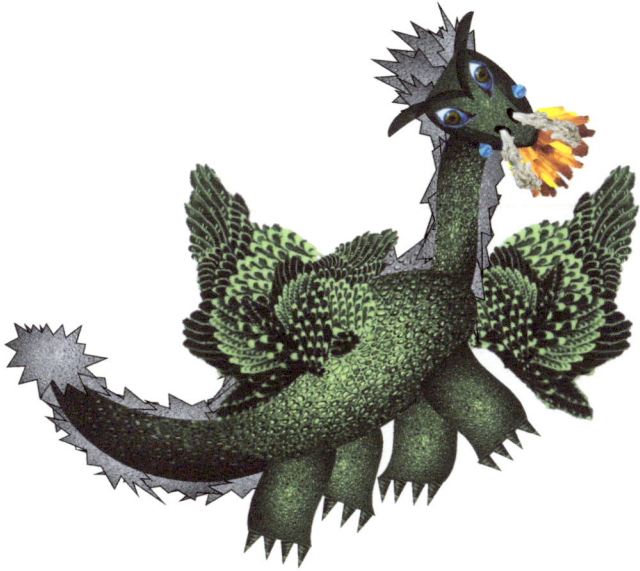

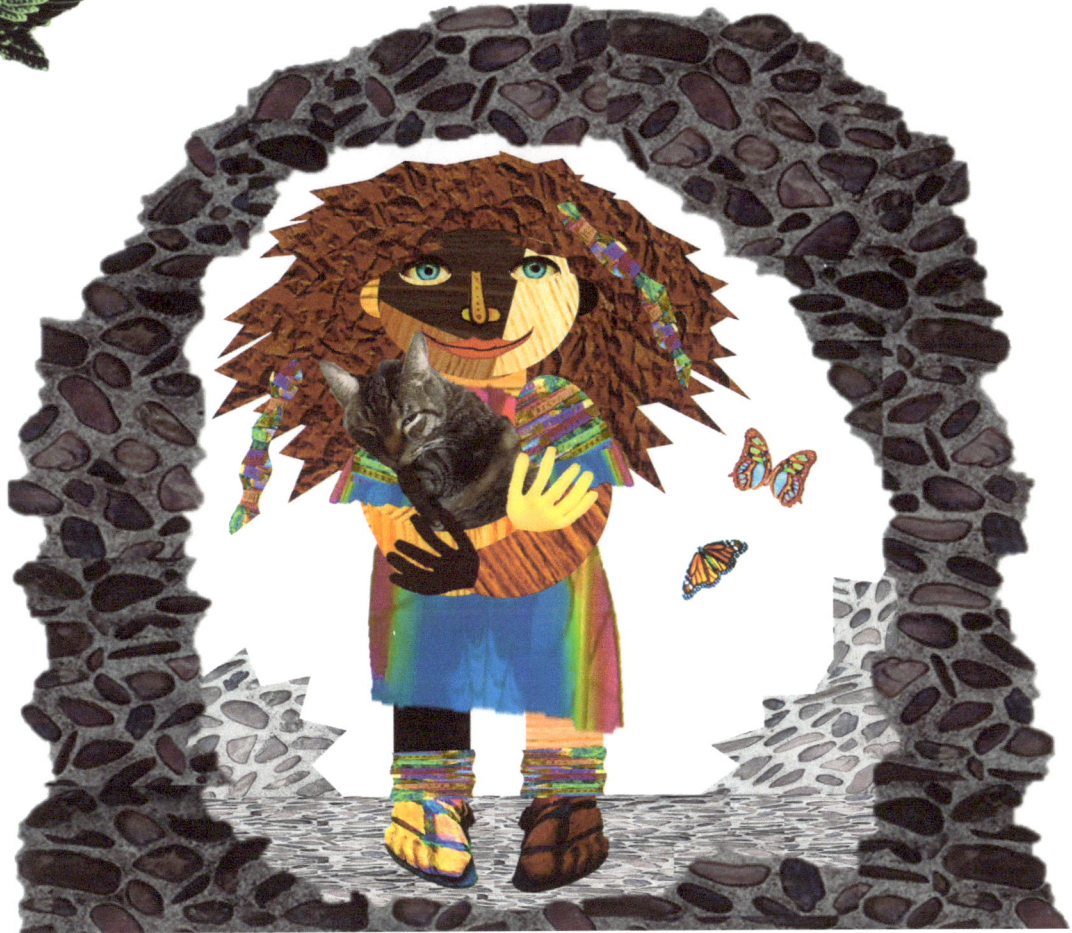

No, children,
I will not teach you about your power
or the power of kinship.
I will not enrobe you in my embrace
or plant kindling inside your spirits
to stoke your fires if they wane.
I will not stitch joy to your songs
or beautiful to your names
so they all become synonyms for one another—
so I can be certain that you will
*never* forget who you are.

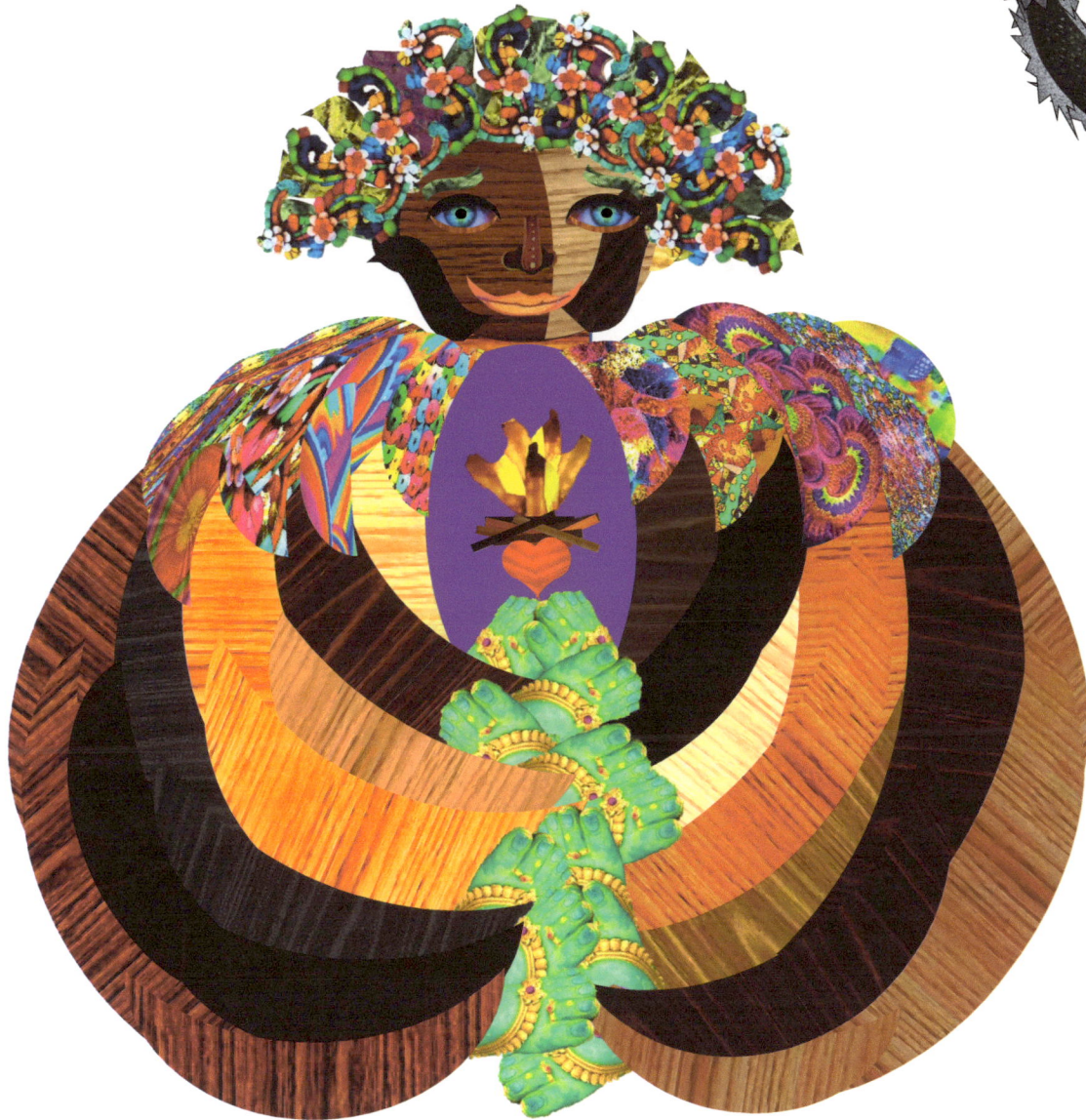

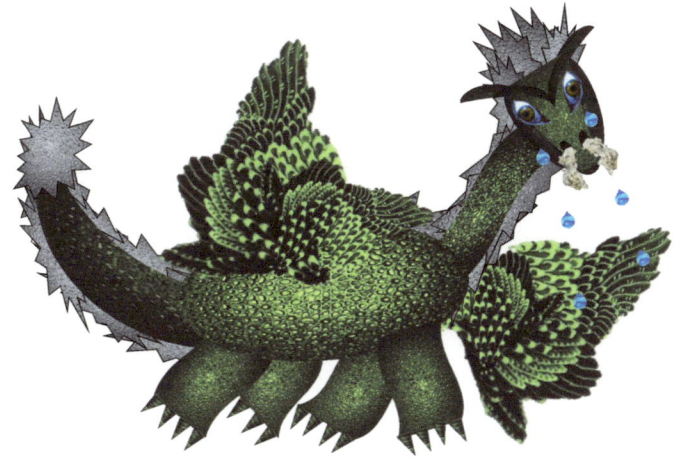

No, my beloved companion in flight,
I will not be here to greet the future
when your path crosses mine,
when fire meets fire
and thunder heralds the news, loud and clear,
so the most distant lightning bolt
and furthest star will hear:
'Rejoice, sisters and brothers of light!
More radiance has just been born!'

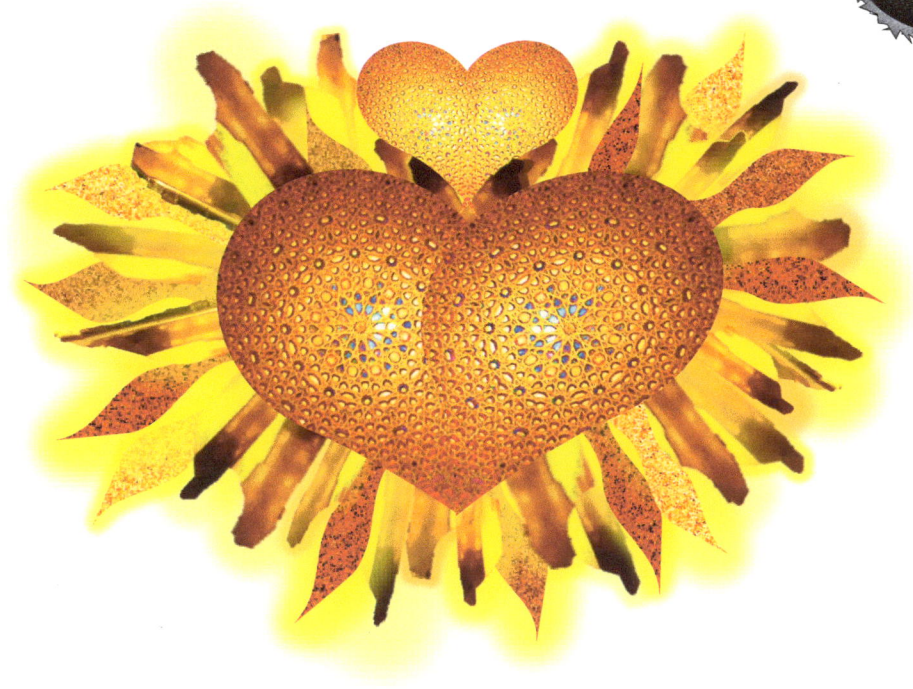

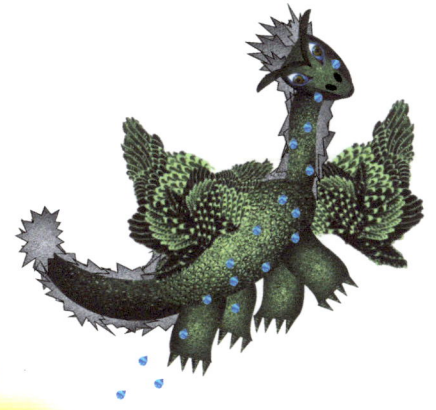

*No.*

I will not be light or laughter or union
or participant in the tenderest acts of love,
for
today
is
my day
to
die."

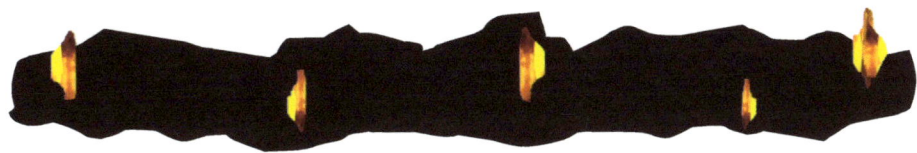

*The new normal.*

Those words set the old normal
shrieking with laughter as it
sharpens blades, loads guns,
stretches its filthy hands and merciless weapons
into tomorrow after tomorrow after tomorrow
while it forewarns through smirking lips,
"My replacement will make you miss me."

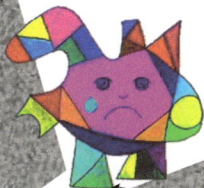

## The new normal.

The phrase doesn't set me counting the days
with a song of tra la la in my heart
because soon everything will be as it was,
except, of course,
for one more layer of masks,

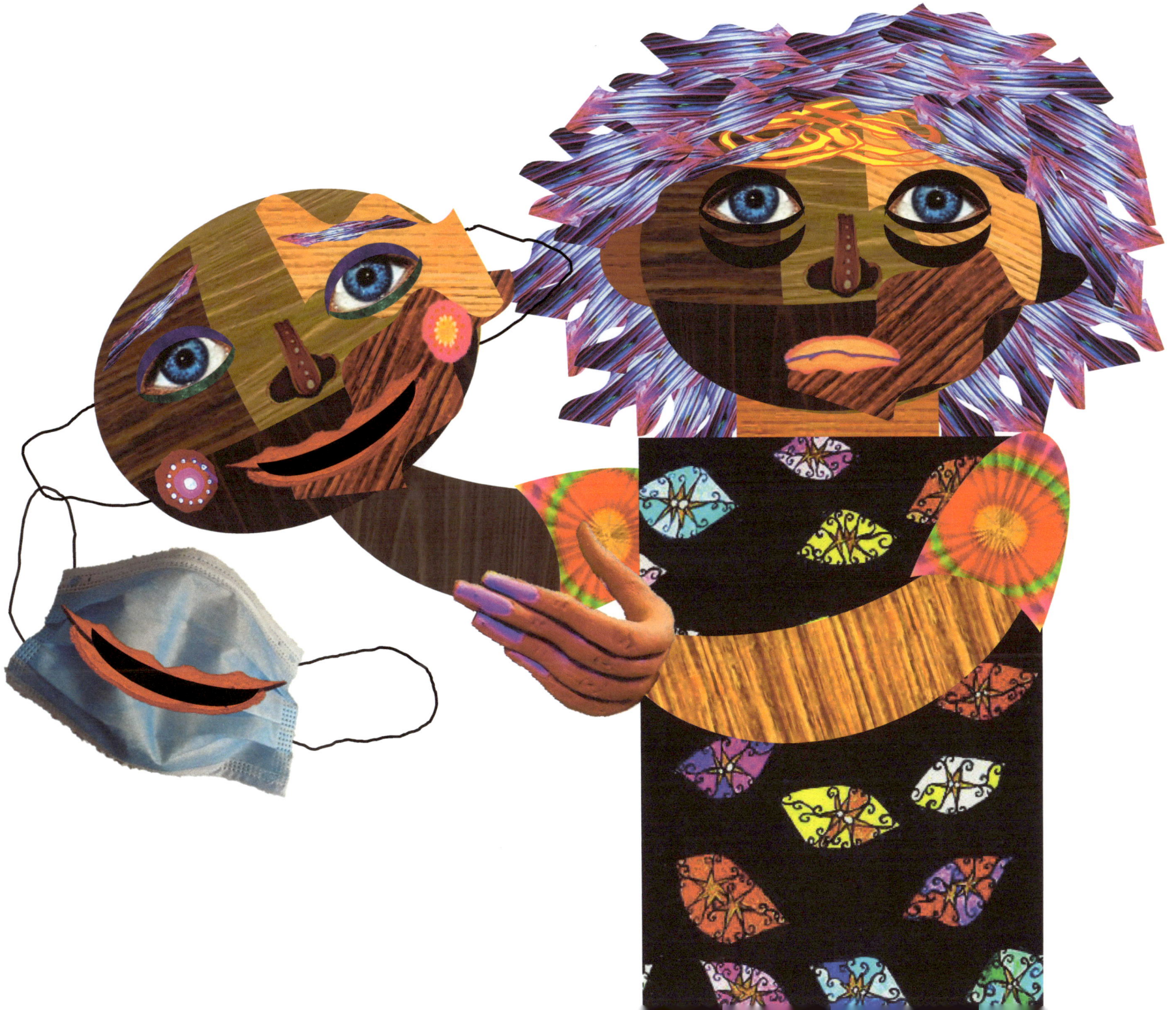

and distance pledging
with fingers crossed behind its back:
"I will save lives."

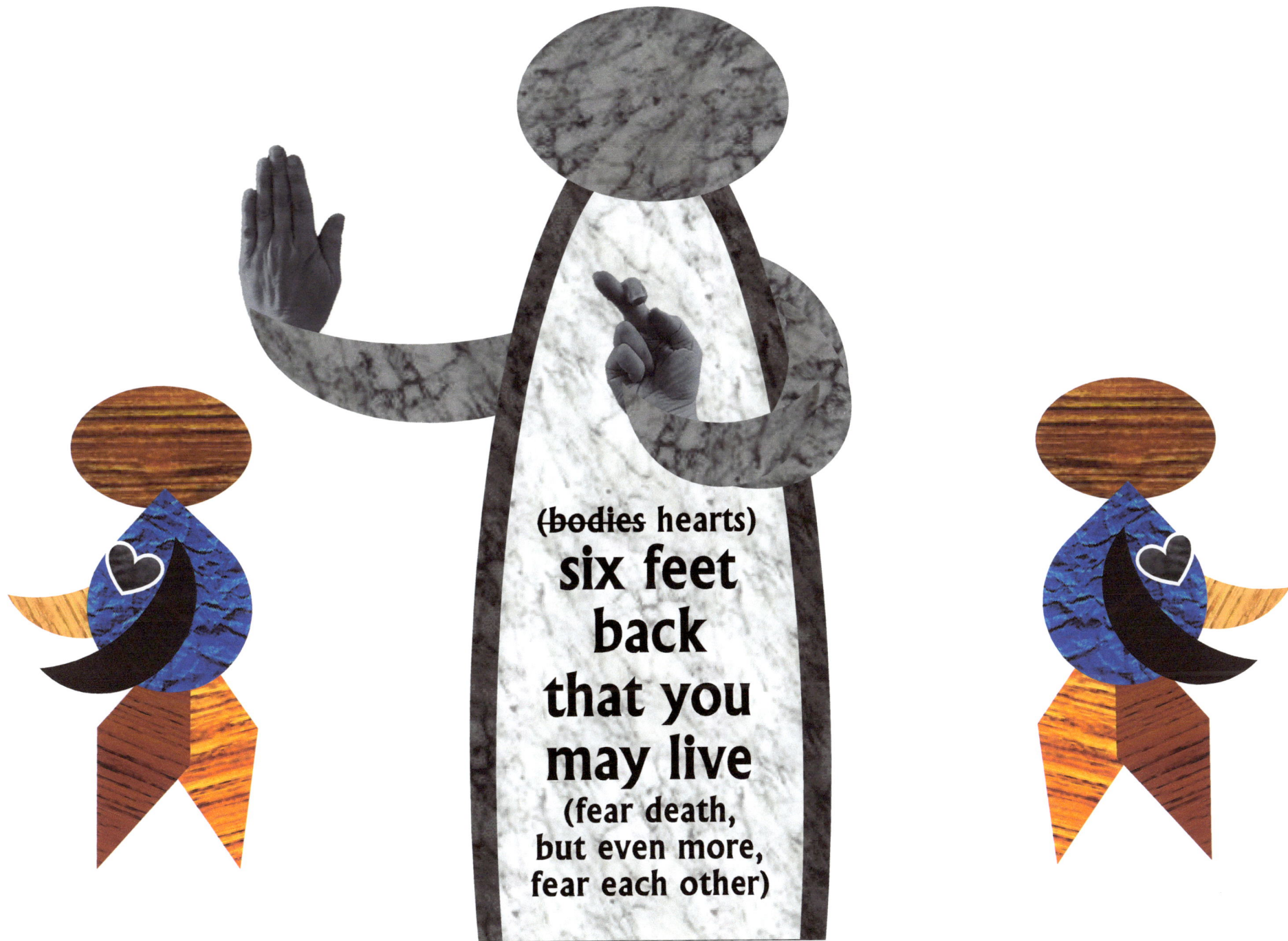

(bodies hearts)

# six feet
# back
# that you
# may live

(fear death,
but even more,
fear each other)

Instead,
the new normal bids me sit at its feet
as it sheds its disguise and reads an old proclamation
with a fresh layer of ink:
"*Different* will suffer consequences.
The outcasts will remain *cast out!*"

Do unto others
as you would
NEVER
want done
unto you.

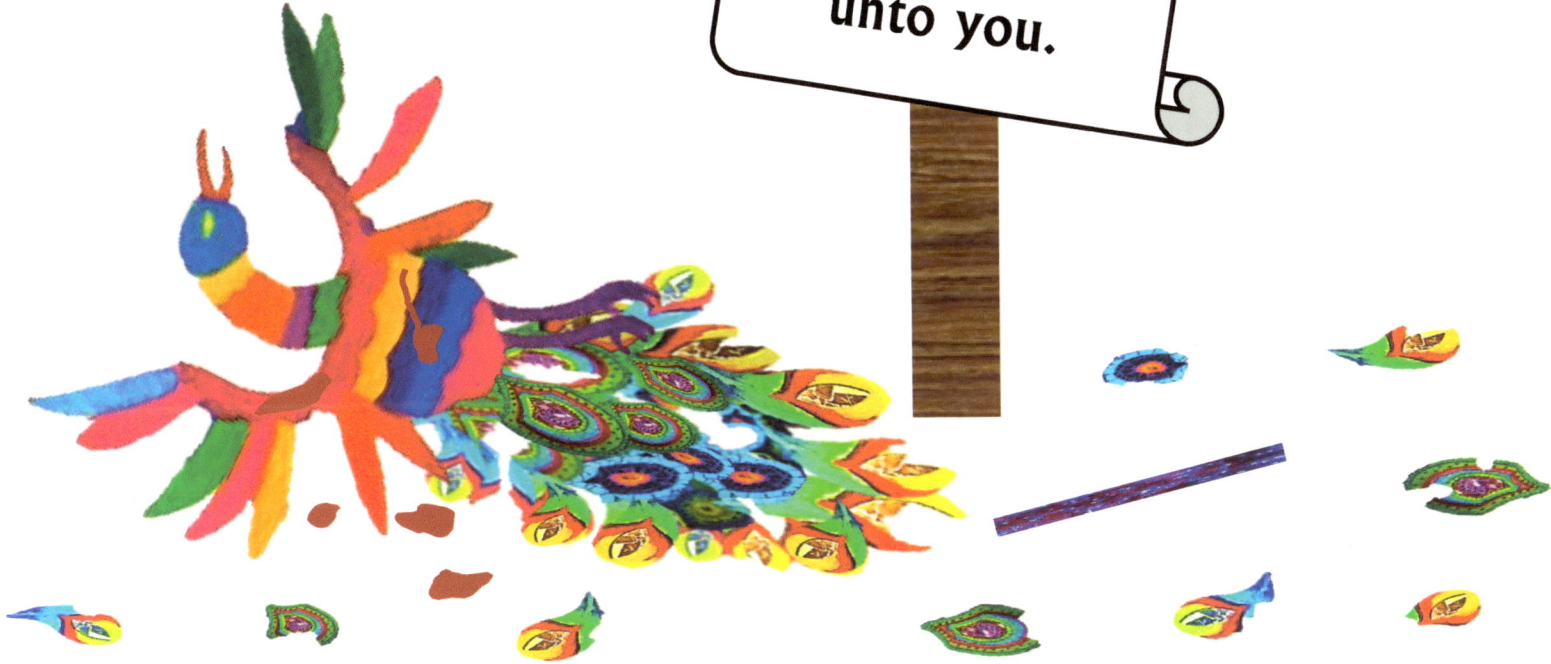

The new normal shushes me back
to the silence I came from;
back to the days when I believed my voice
was something I needed permission to use;
back to the certainty that my words
were unworthy of being heard;
back to songs that writhed unsung
and gifts that died ungiven.

R.I.P.
W.I.P.
WRITHE
IN
PAIN

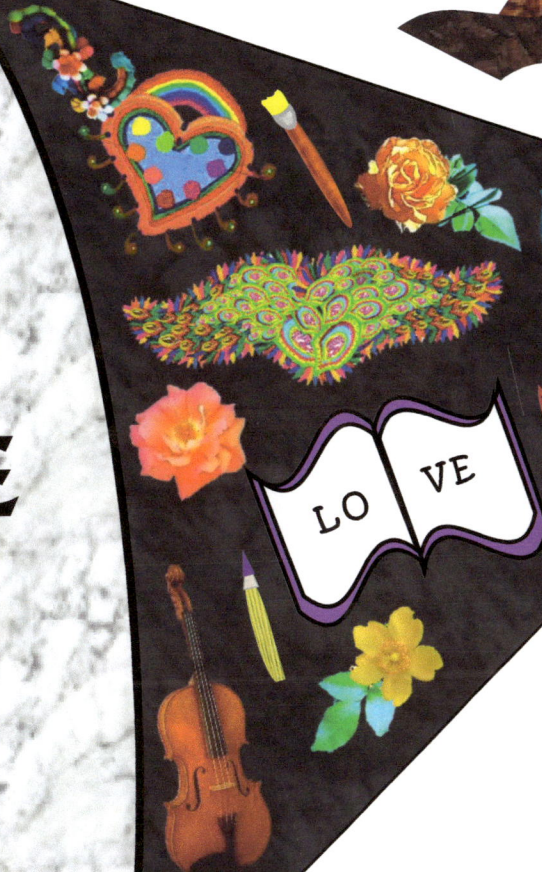

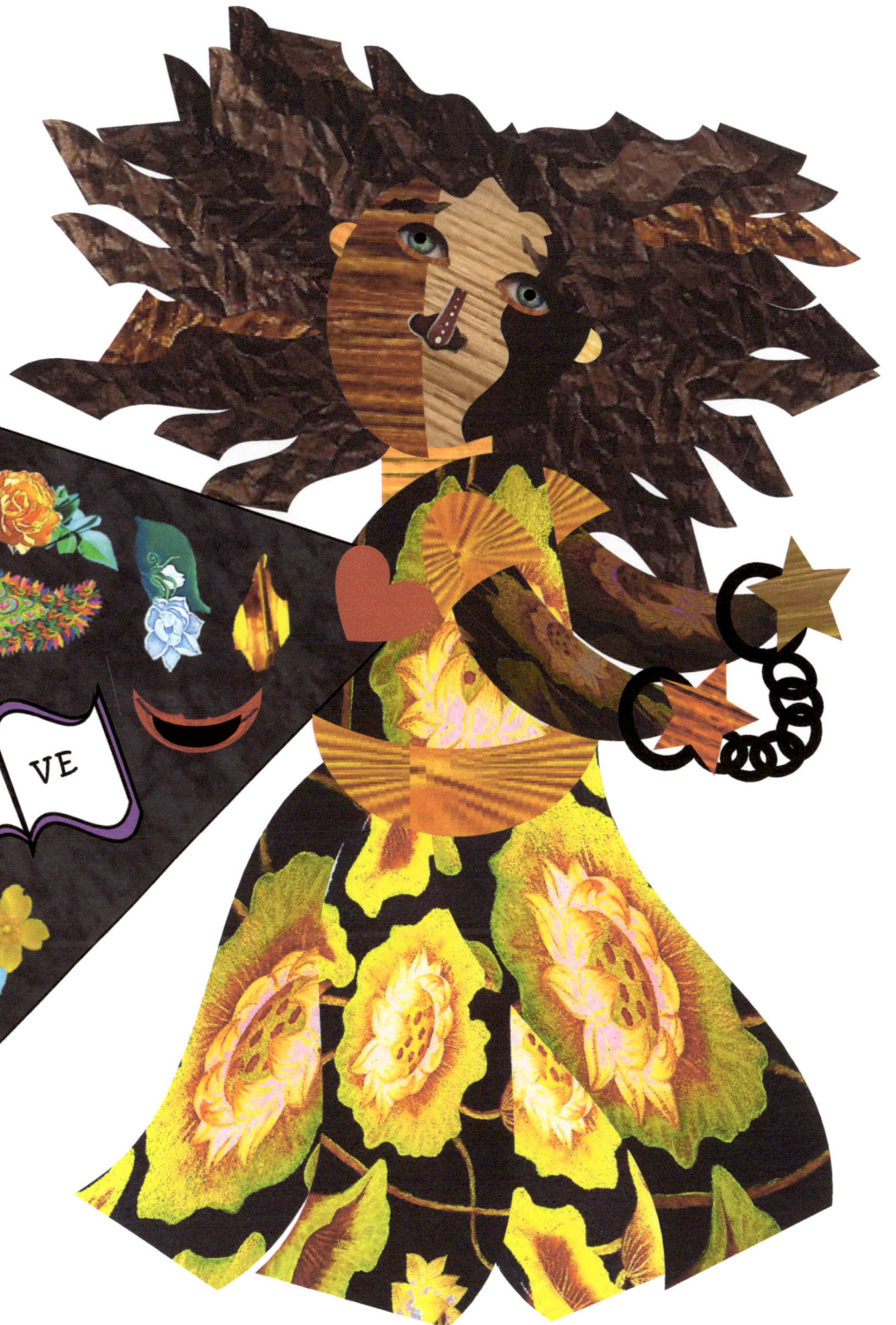

LO VE

The new normal makes me fear that
things will continue to be misnamed:
the illogical, senseless, and unjustifiable
forever stripped of their prefixes and suffixes;

# Justifiable

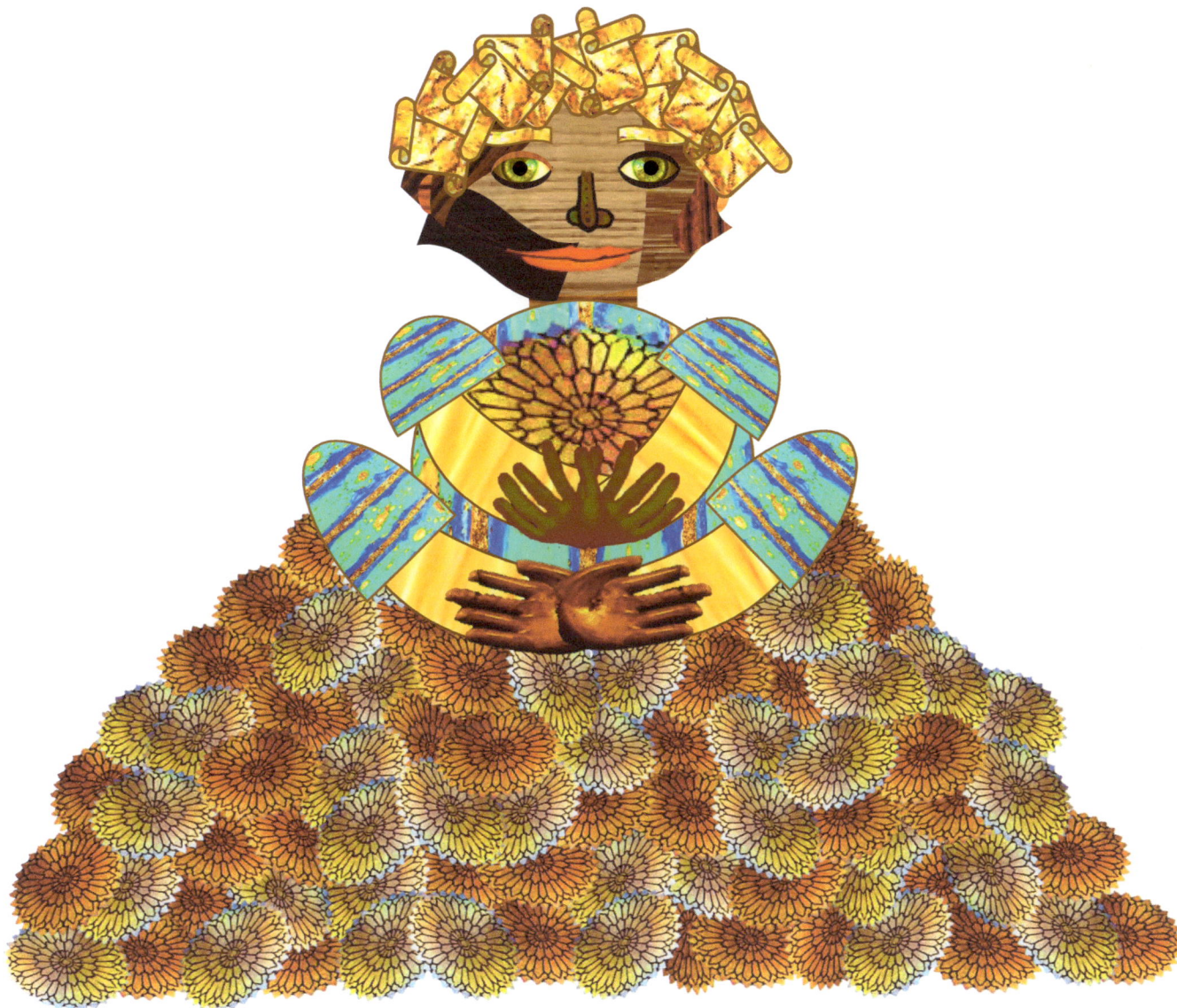

un

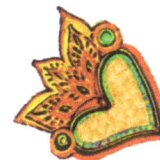

ailing spirits severed from the sanity
that the correct words restore.

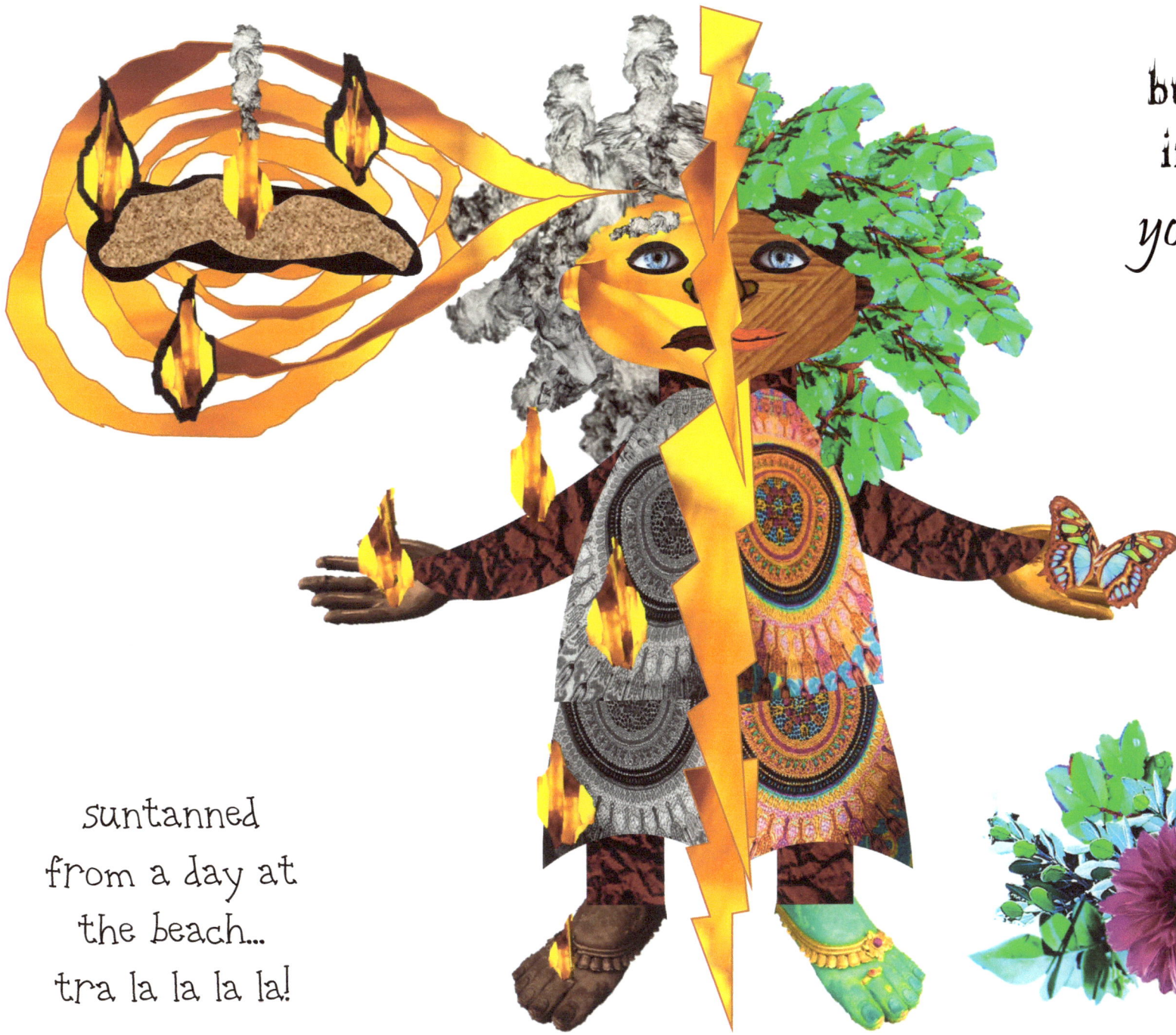

nearly
burned alive
in a blaze...
*you will heal*

suntanned
from a day at
the beach...
tra la la la la!

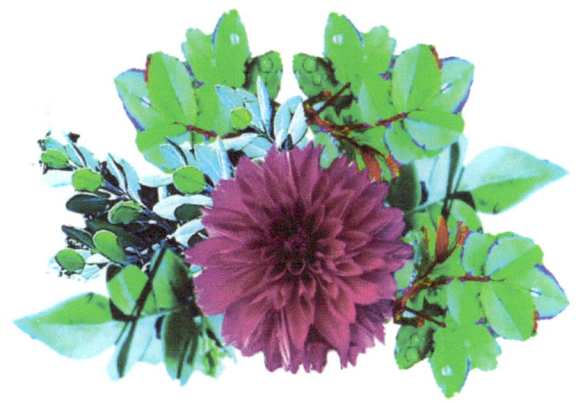

And so...

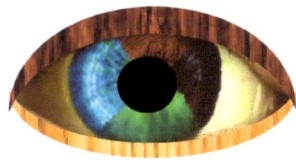

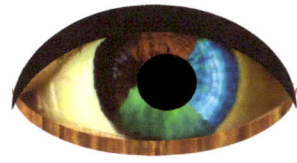

War crimes will still be forbidden
but war still allowed.

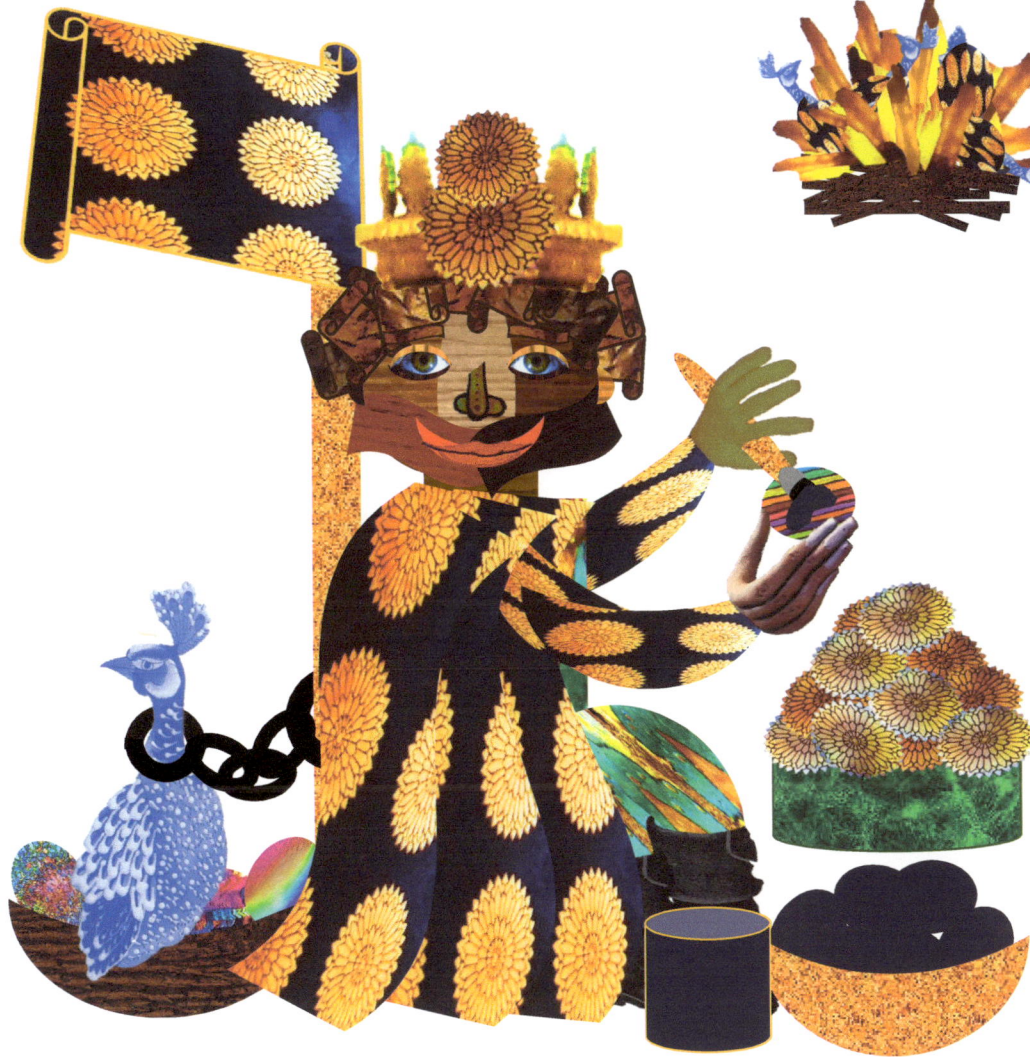

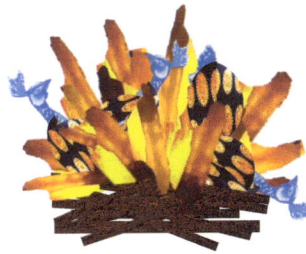

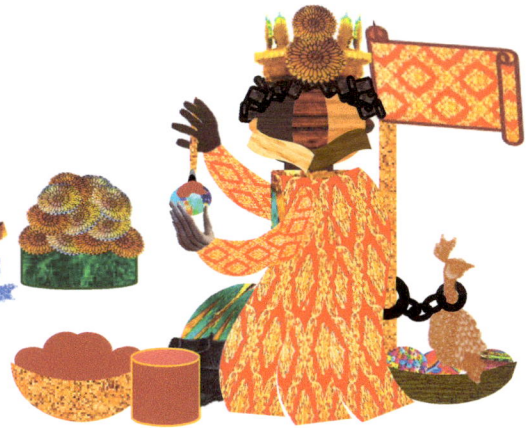

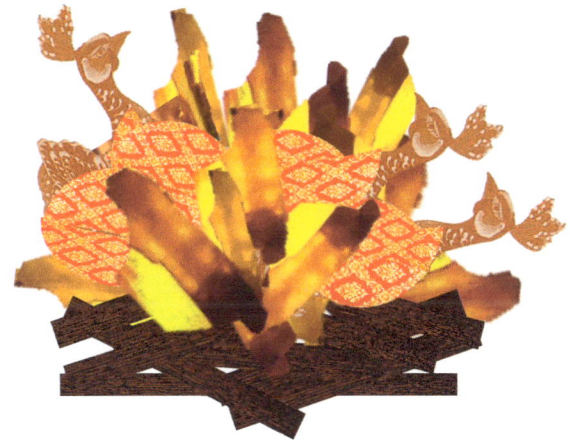

In the name of humanity,
we will still speak of the economy
and swear that privileging the second
will aid the first.

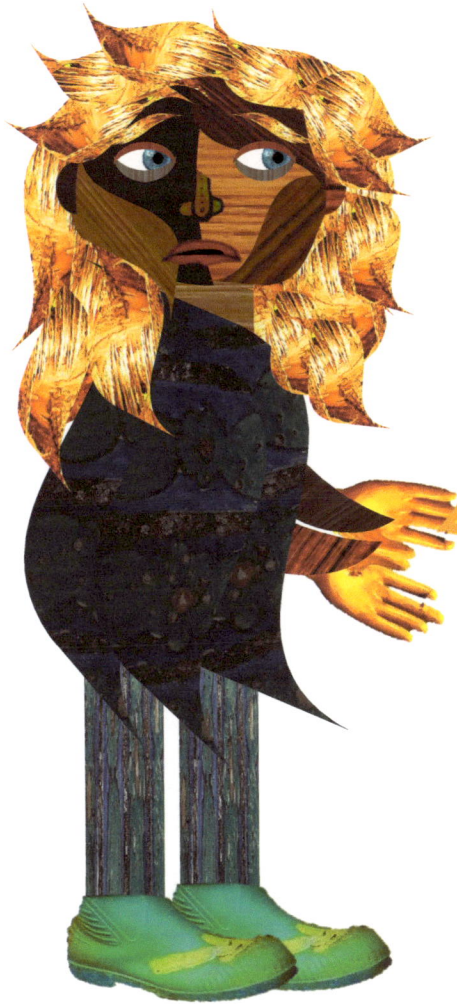

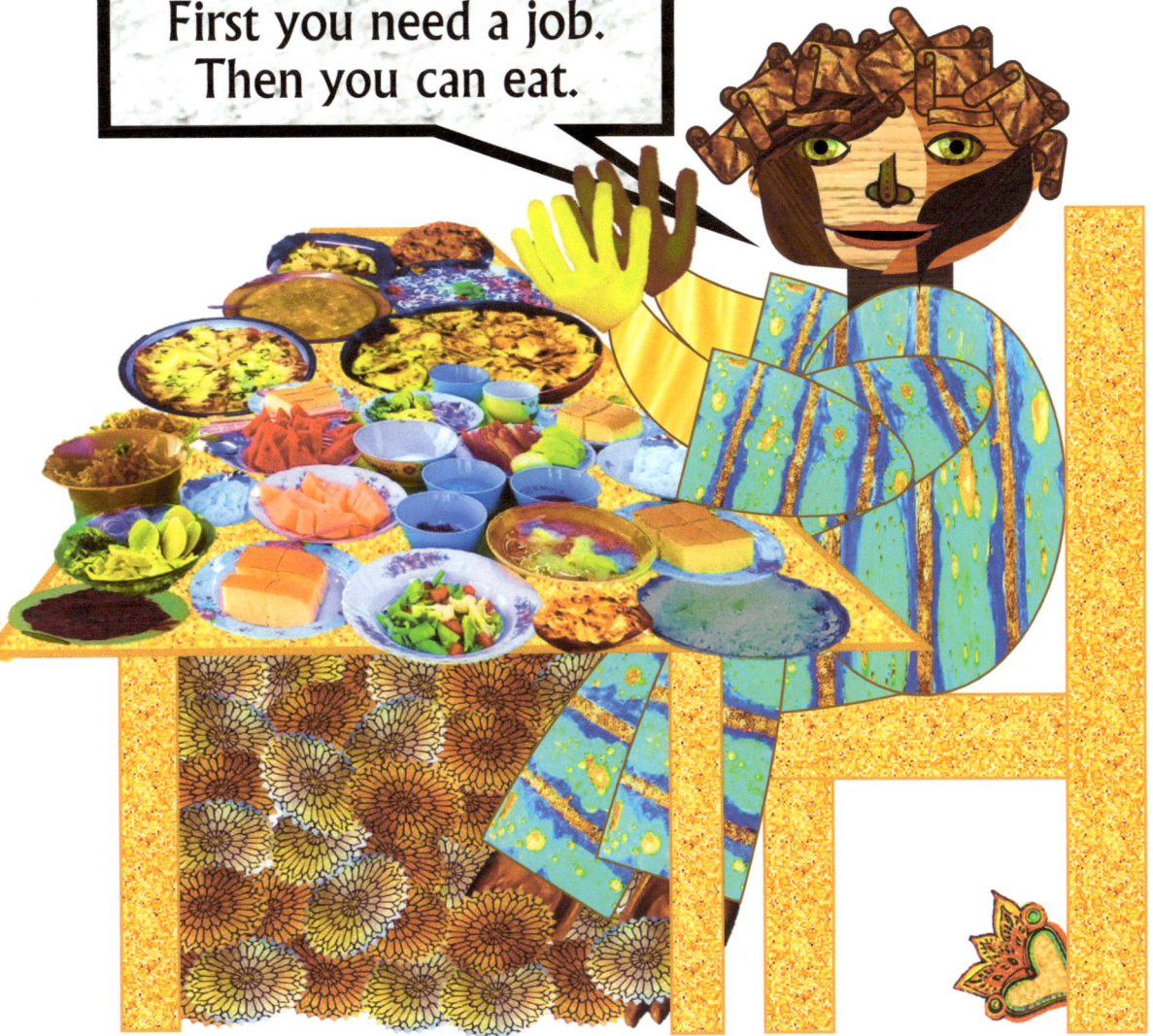

In the temples of fear,
we will still beseech power
to favor us over others.

## Uniforms/Gowns/Robes/Ceremonial Garments

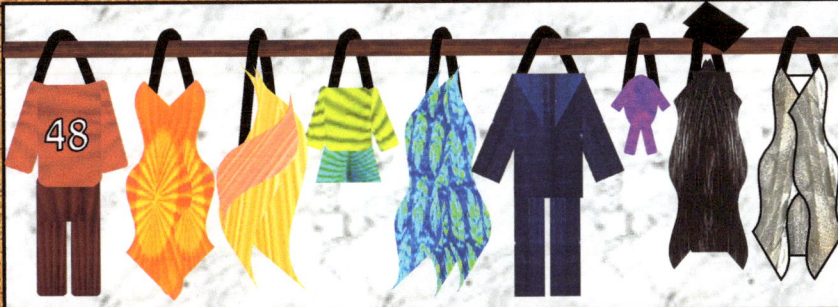

48

**Start here.**

Be afraid.

## Prayers

Please let _____ _____ _____ instead of _____.
(column 1) (column 2) (column 3) (column 4)

| COLUMN 1 | COLUMN 2 | COLUMN 3 | COLUMN 4 |
|---|---|---|---|
| • me | • be | • the best | • him |
| • us | • win | • the first | • her |
| • my/our child/ren | • get | • the gold | • them |
| • my/our family | • receive | • the game | • her _____ |
| • my/our team | • have | • the job | • his _____ |
| • my/our school | • _____ | • rich | • their _____ |
| • my/our group | • _____ | • Your protection | • _____ |
| • my/our people | • _____ | • Your favor | • _____ |
| • my/our country | • _____ | • Your love | • _____ |
| • my/our _____ | • _____ | • _____ | • _____ |

In the systems of instruction,
indoctrination
will still demand that
education
reward answers

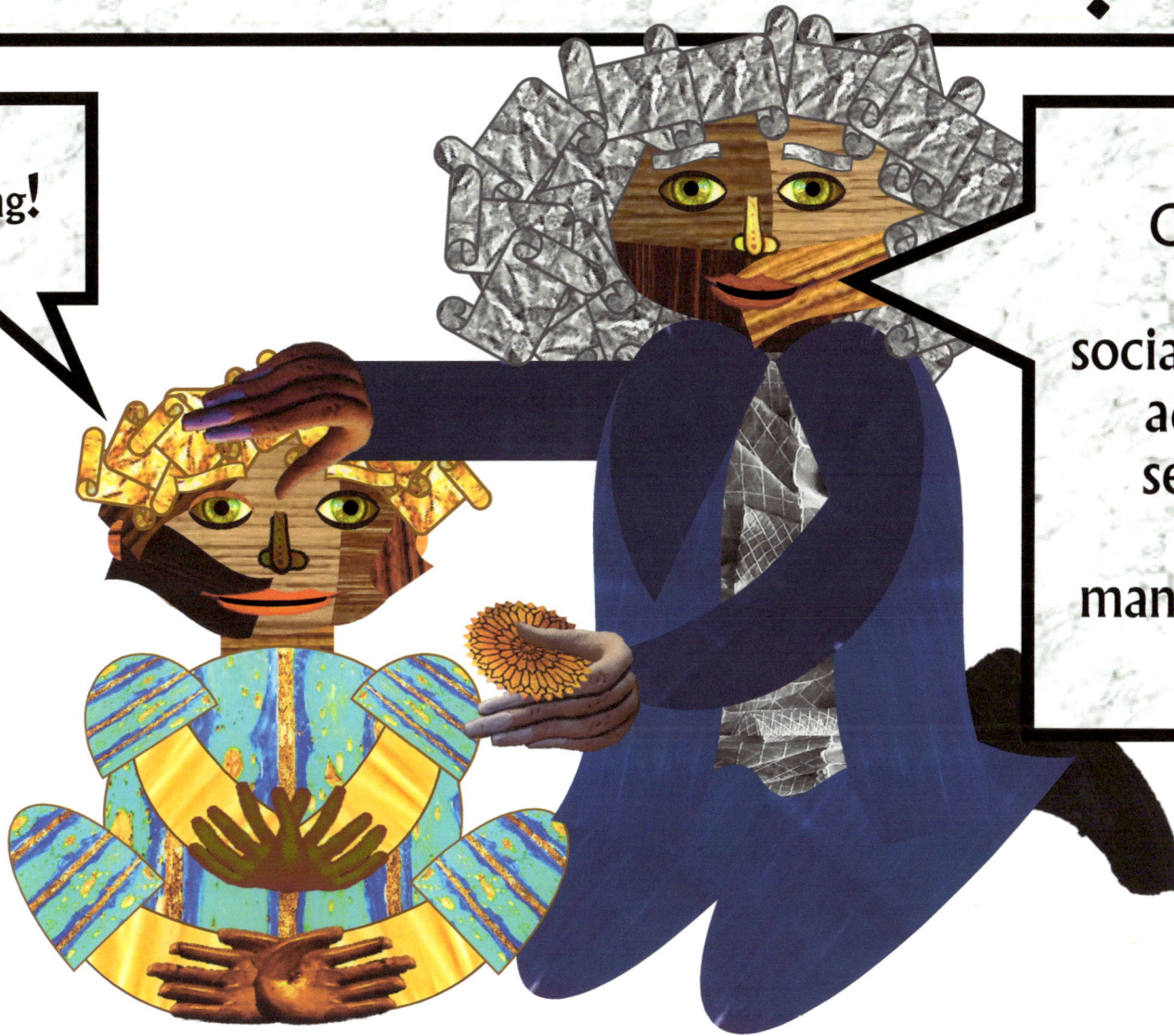

and
punish questions.

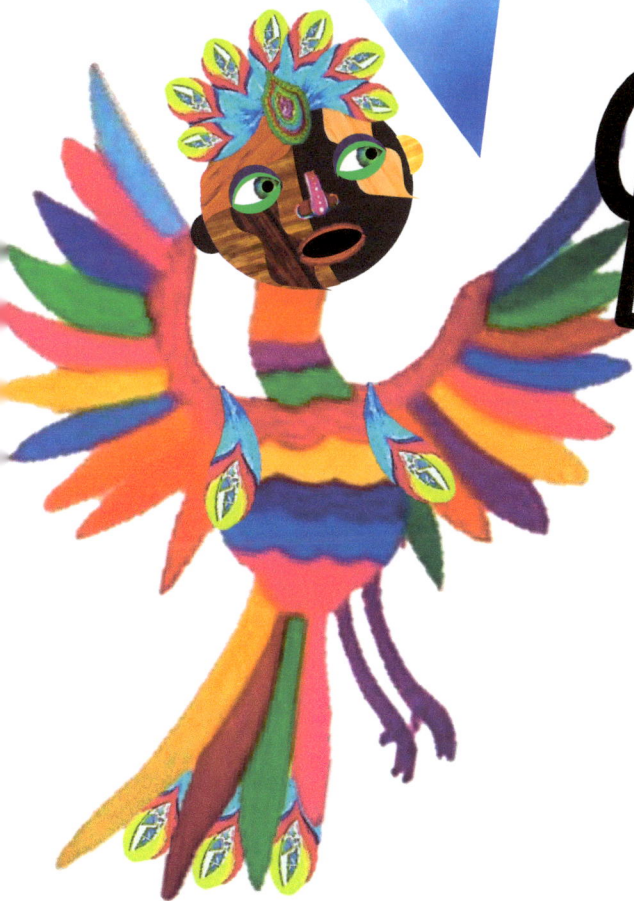

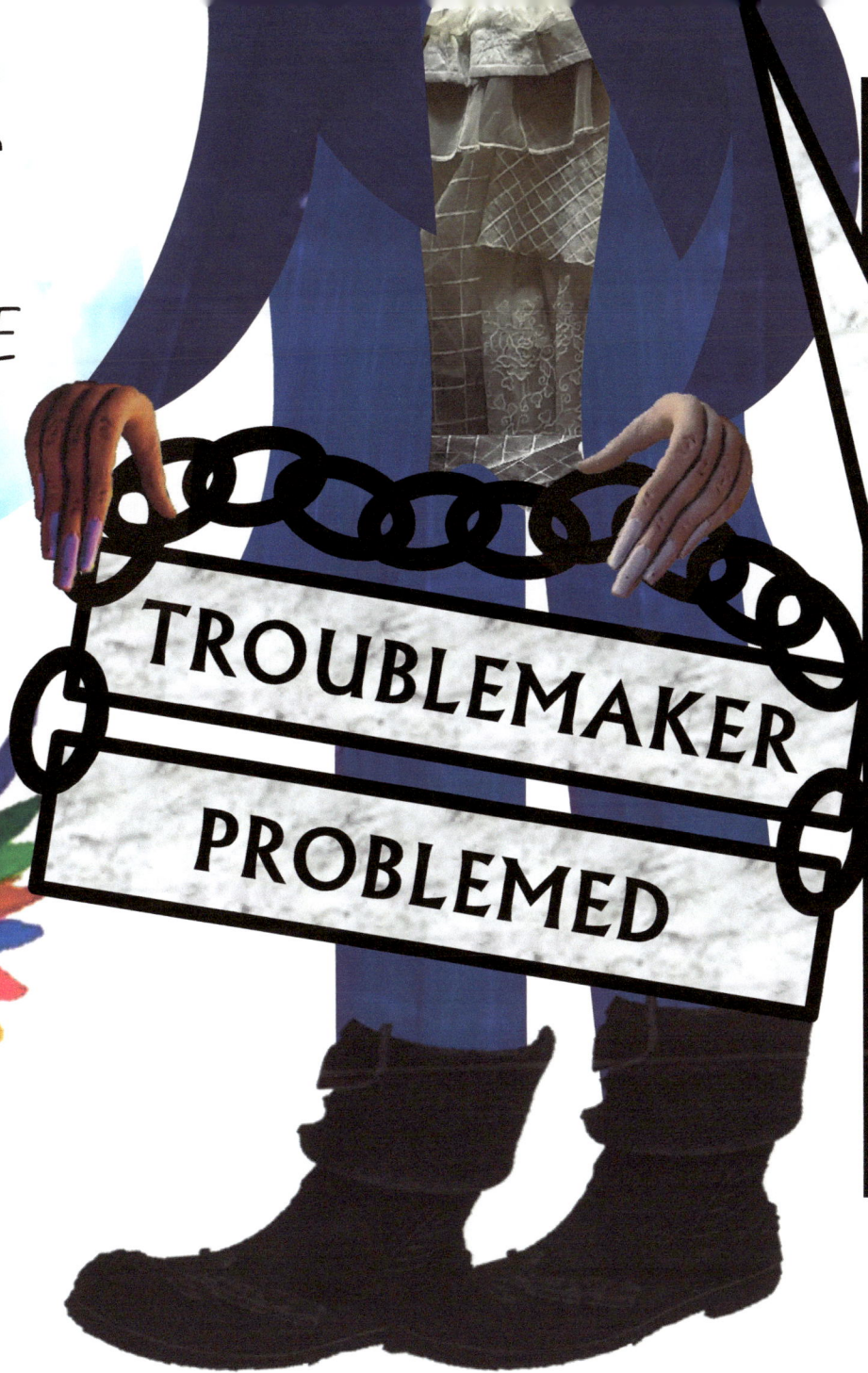

The assaulted will still be convicted
for the atrocities committed against them.

# CRIMES
- hunger
- poverty
- short skirt
- skin color
- love
- existence

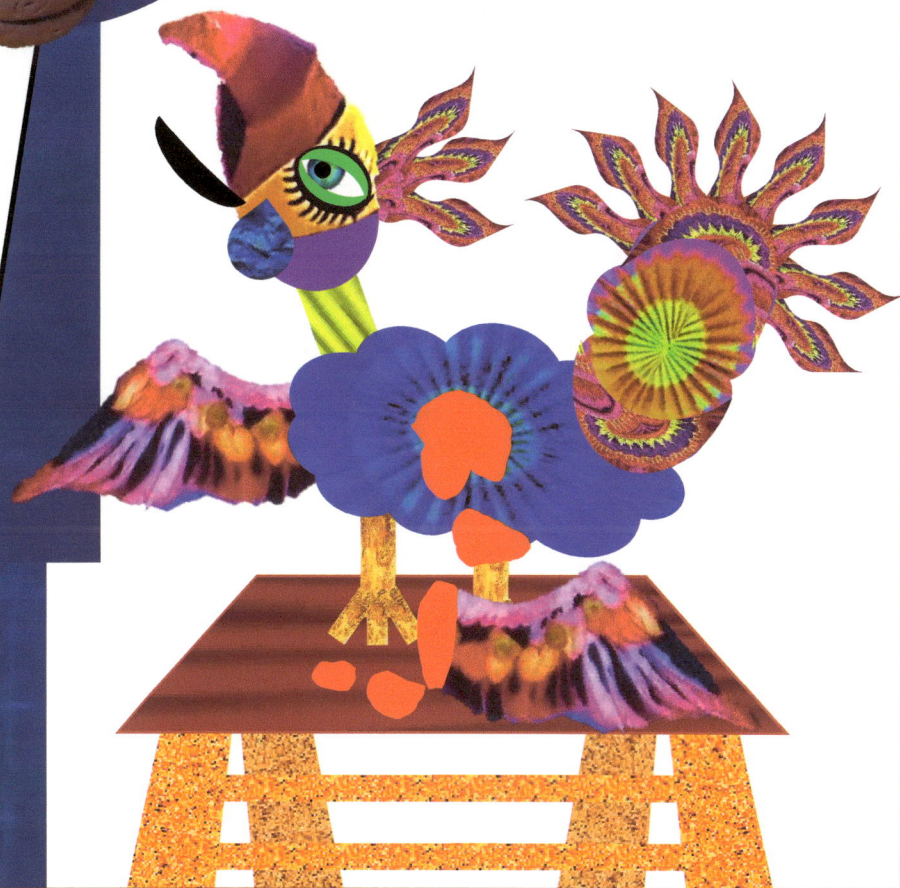

Beauty will still be beaten into a state of amnesia.

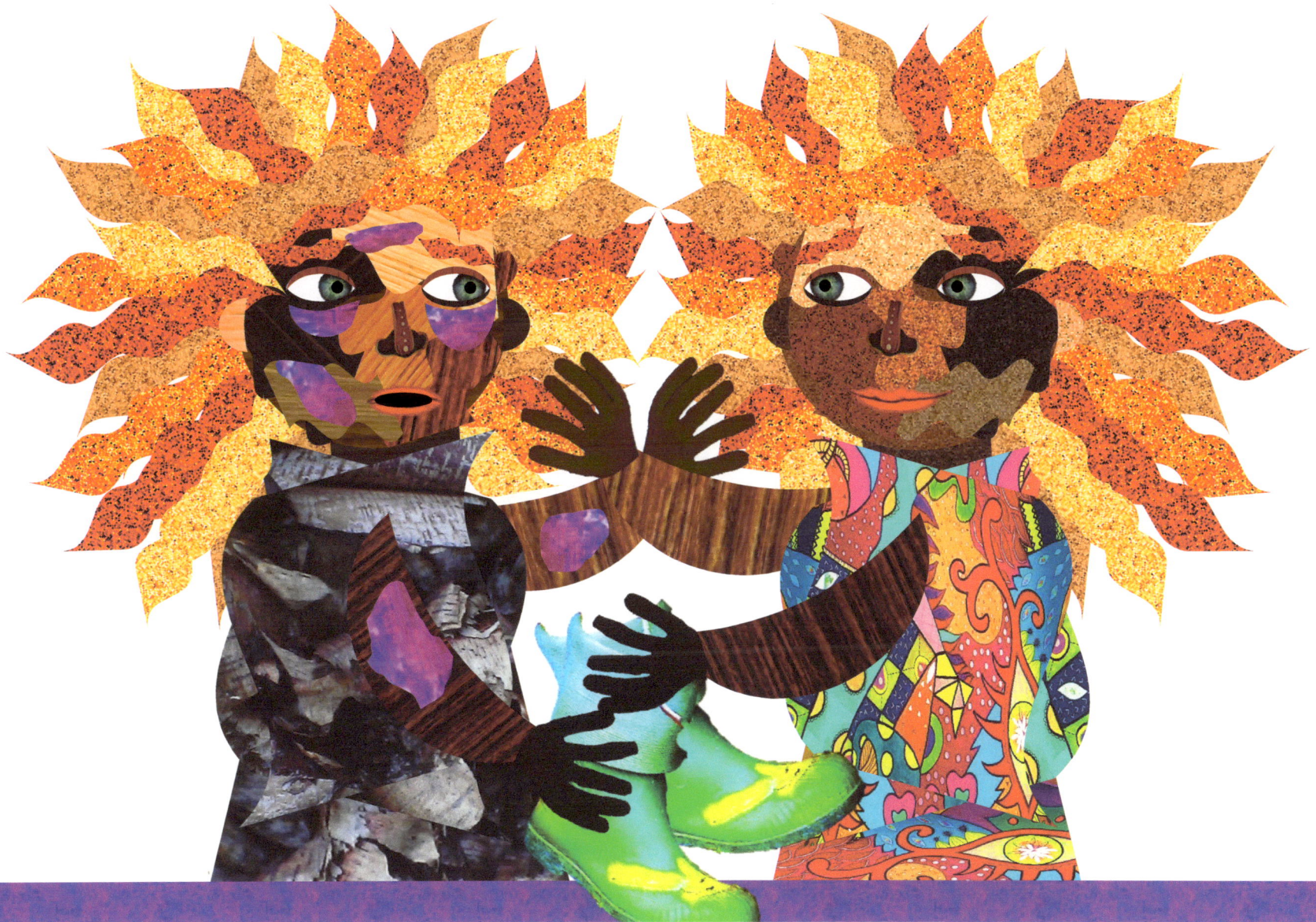

Anguish will still be called weakness
and
symptoms still designated diseases
as the root causes of suffering are buried in
deeper
and
deeper
graves.

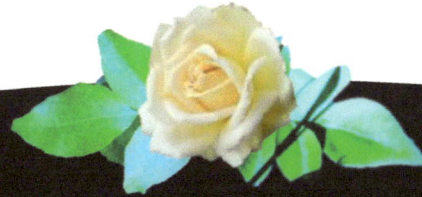

R.I.P.
Dear
Disturbed
Soul

R
Dis

suicide

mental illness

MURDER

trauma          cruelty          violence

dehumanization     abuse          injustice

bullying       loneliness        poverty

pressure     disempowerment      exclusion

systemic oppression      fear      hatred

The earth will still grieve
as her forests are felled and glaciers melted;
as her water is syphoned away
from those dying of thirst;
and as her laws of liberty are repeatedly repealed,
and swimming seas and crossing fields

remain crimes.

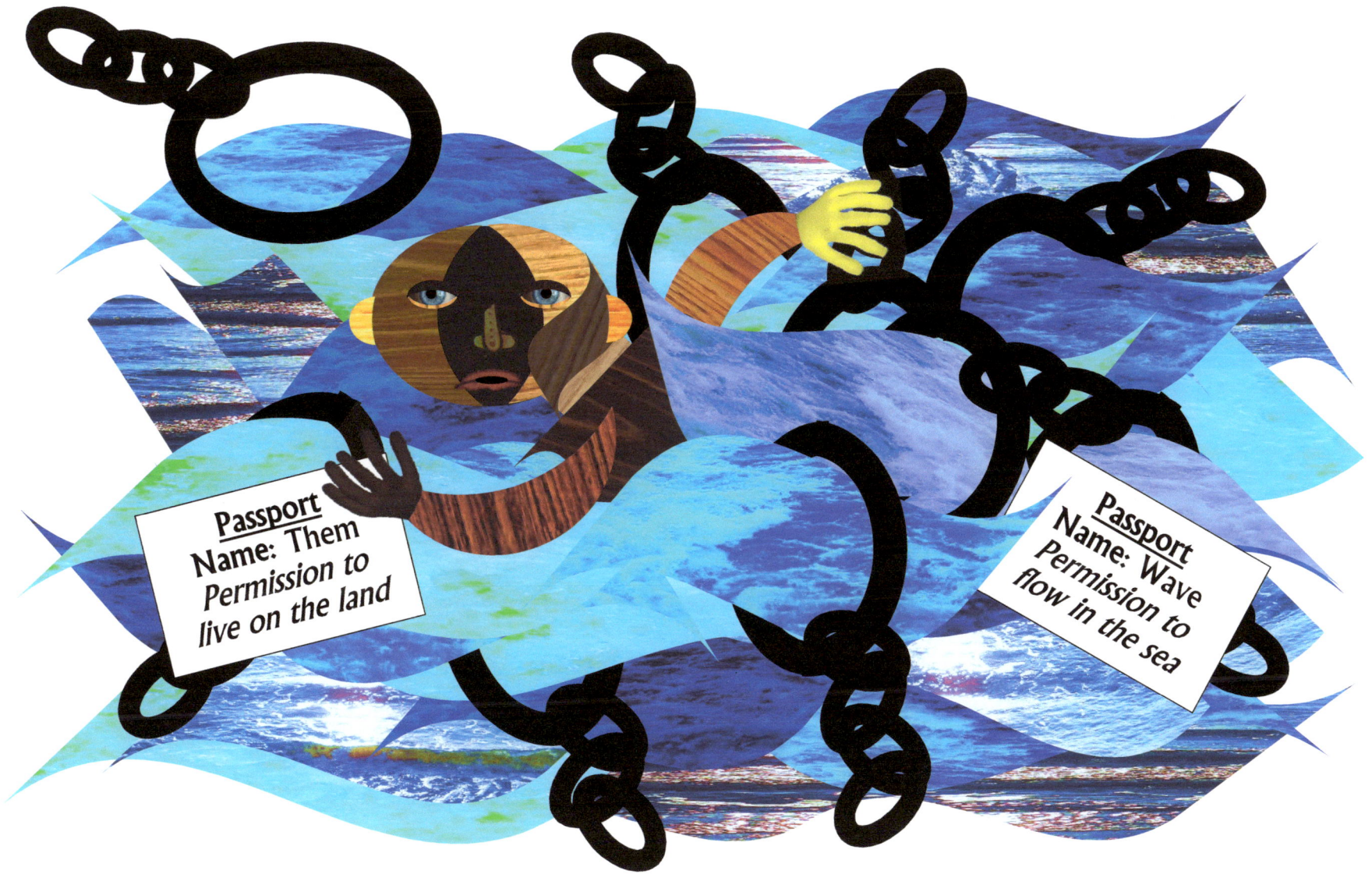

Passport
Name: Them
Permission to
live on the land

Passport
Name: Wave
Permission to
flow in the sea

Love will still cry out,
"What have you done with the purpose I gave you?"
as it attempts to suture wounds into scars
with needles worn dull from never-ending use.

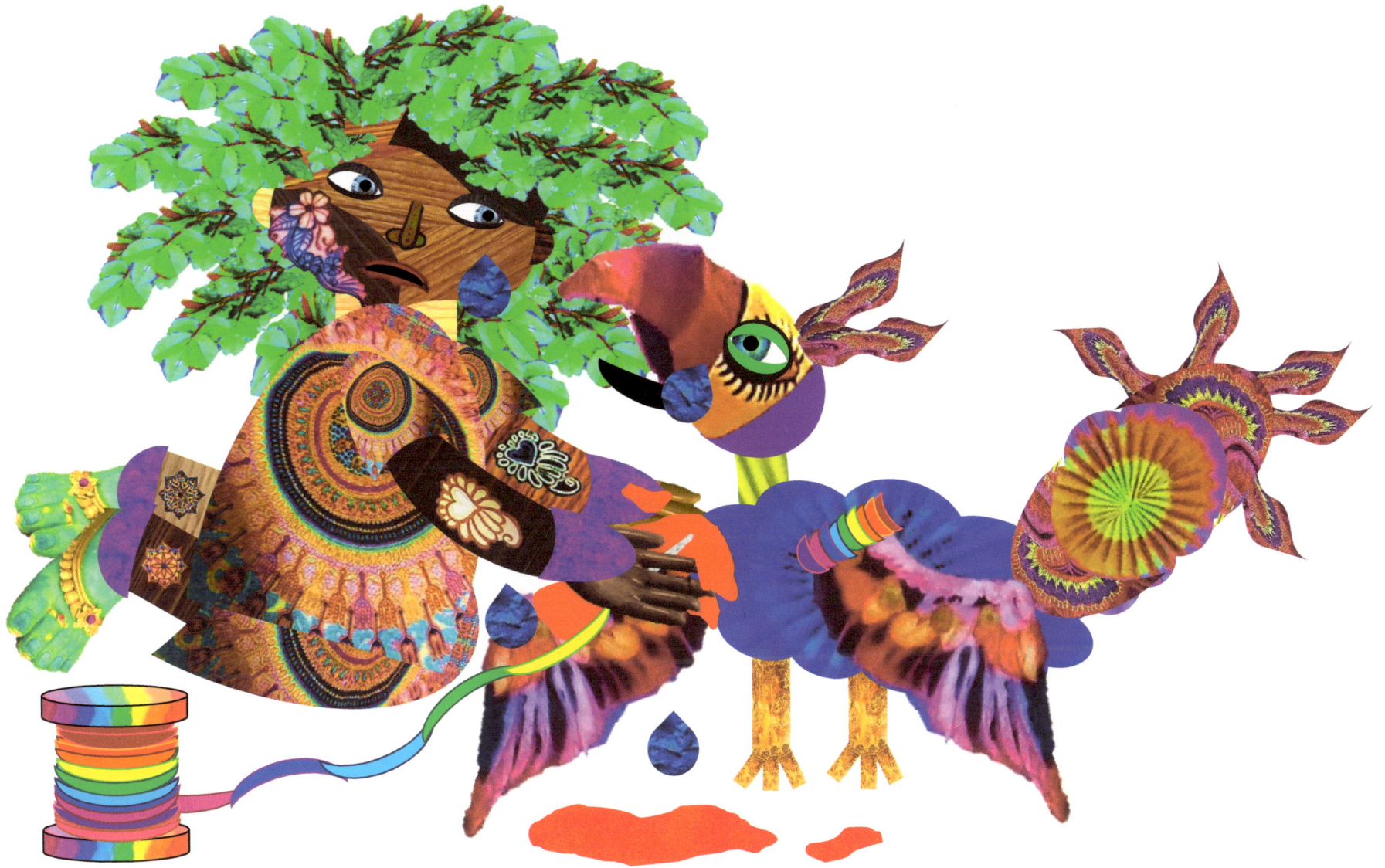

Life will still scream,
"No!" and "Not what I meant!"
as its wildness is tortured and tamed
into narrow, concrete paths
that most everyone is meant to walk or lay,
whatever the case may be,
depending upon the identity and station in life
that a roll of the dice bore them into.

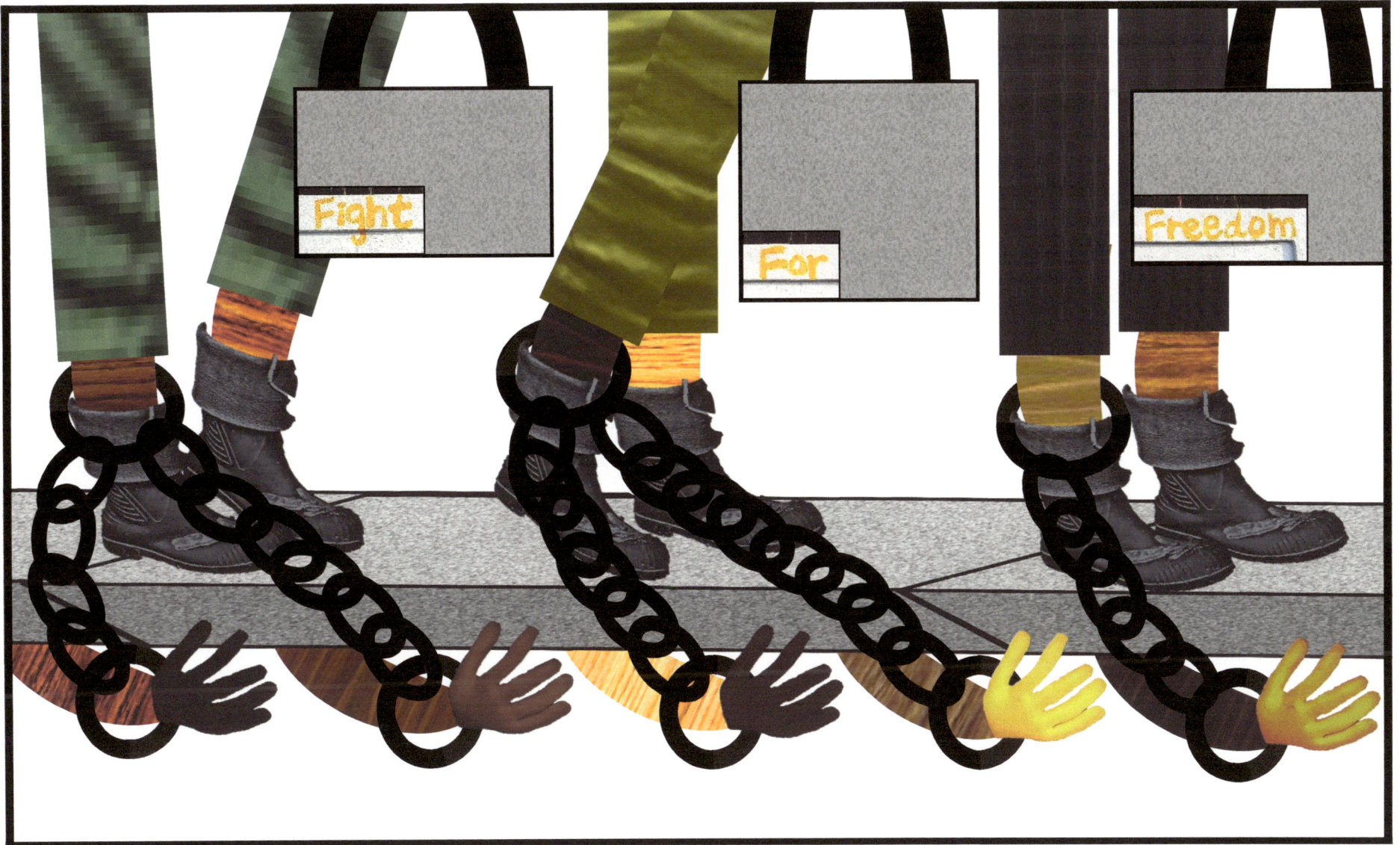

Those who do not or cannot conform
will still be crushed in the fringes
by those who walk with heedless steps
because long ago
they were *taught*
and
they *learned*:
it's eat or be eaten.

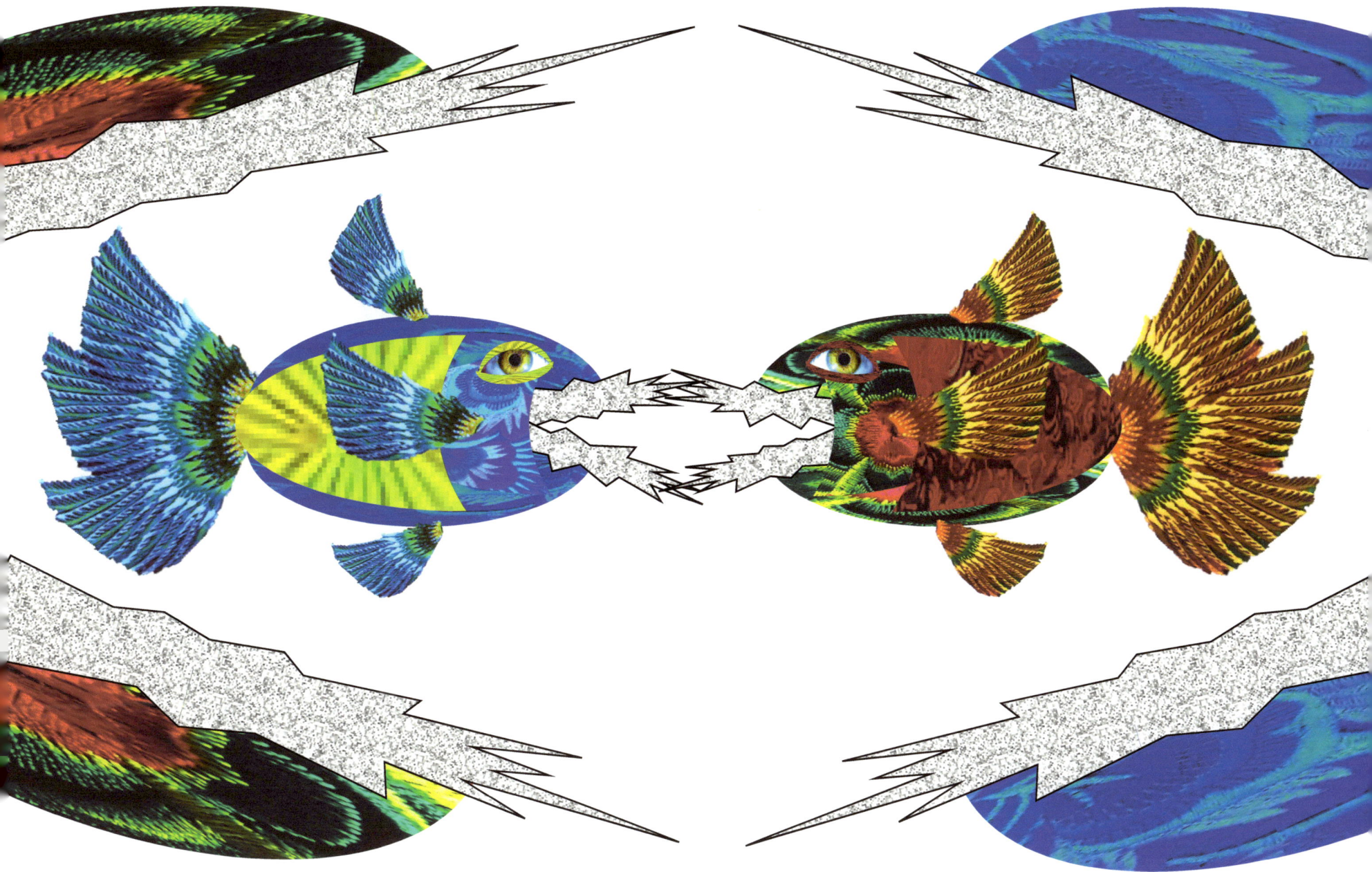

And children will still be forbidden
from staring too long at the sky
because
imagination
can
disrupt
*everything—*
most of all,
normal.

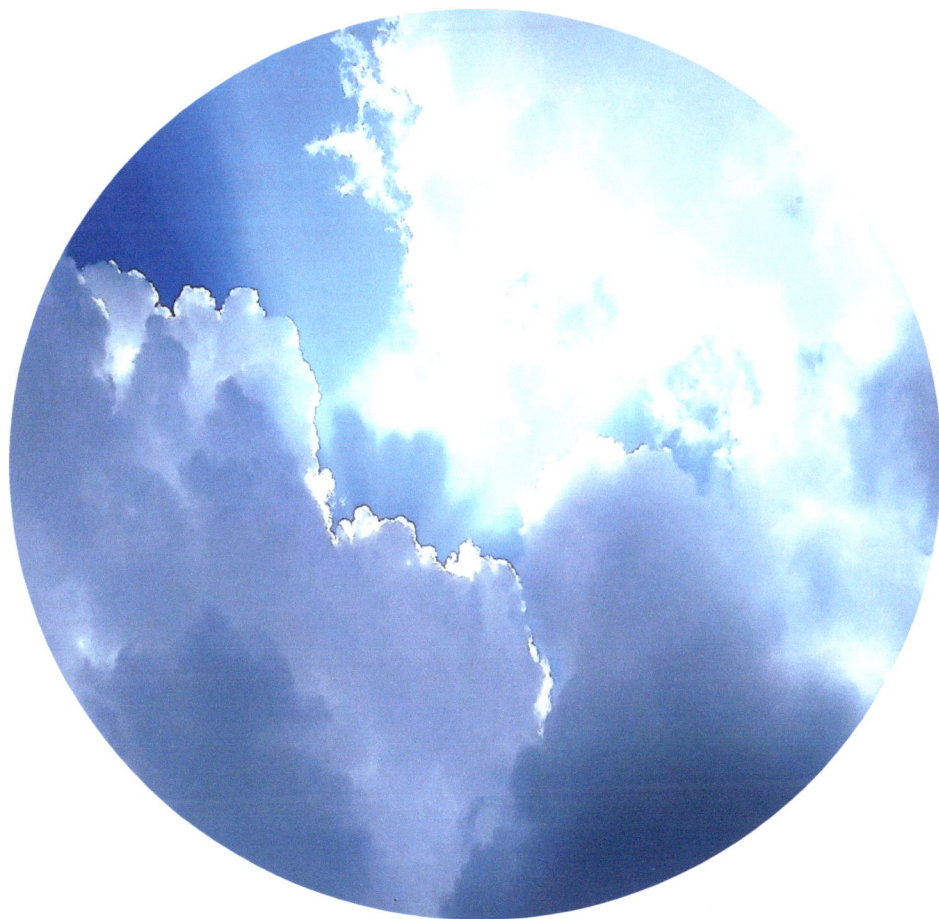

But...

if we wrench our imaginations free
from all that would send them to a silent tomb,
perhaps the new normal can be
an opening instead of a closing.

Perhaps its definition is still up for grabs,
and we who have been shut out and shut down,
we who have been called
*crazy, worthless, abnormal,*

we who have held on to our questions
for dear life
and held on to our lives
with bloody hands,
can have a say in creating a way of life
that does not leave
myriads
wishing
they had never lived at all.

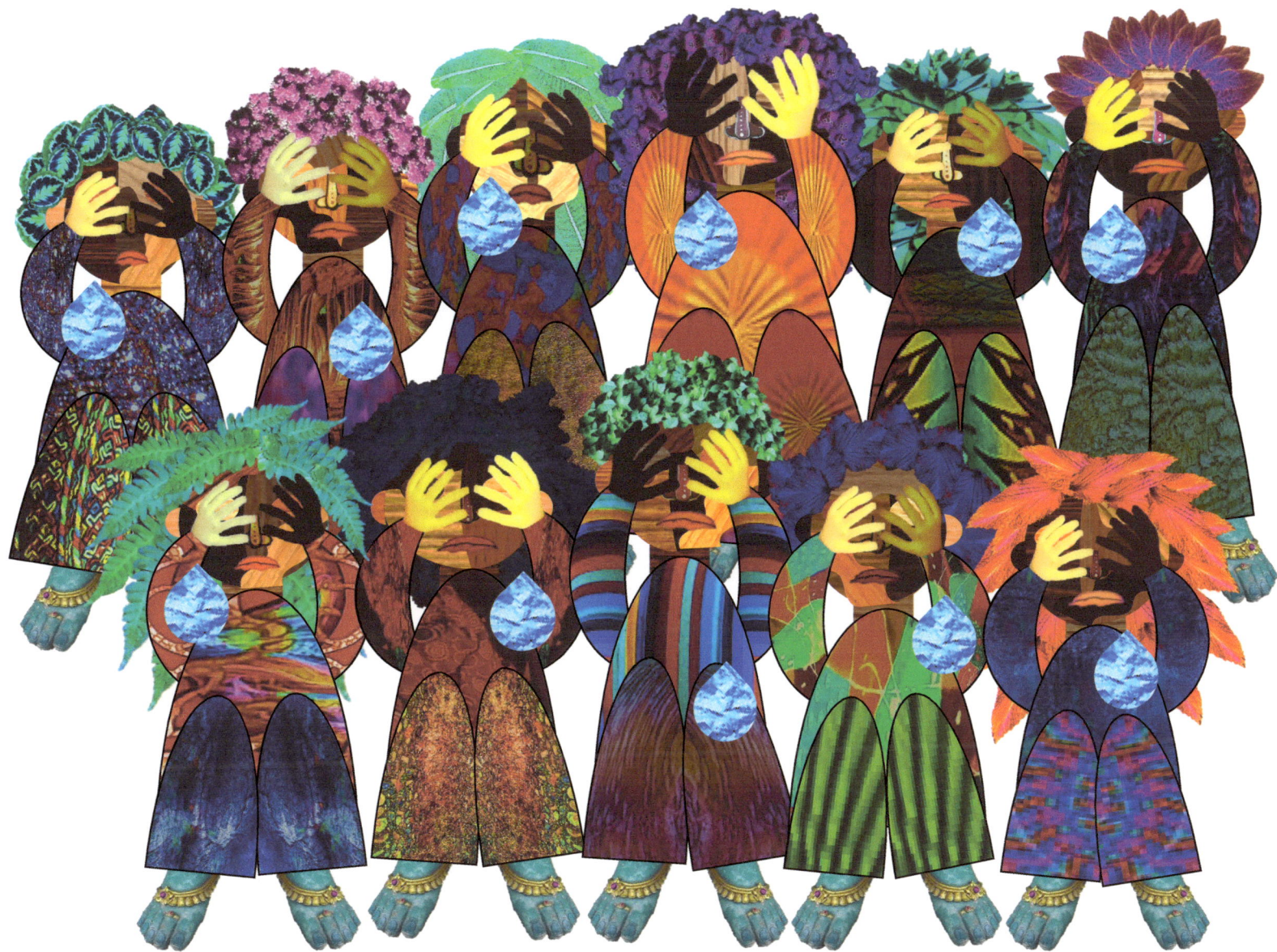

The bedrock of the new normal can be this fact:

We are perfect as we are.

*Not* perfect in the sense that
we are deserving of the vile inheritance
passed down from one generation of
misunderstood and feared to another,
a scorching mark of shame burned so deeply into us
that our spirits wince and
we have bowed our heads and begged apologies
for being ourselves.

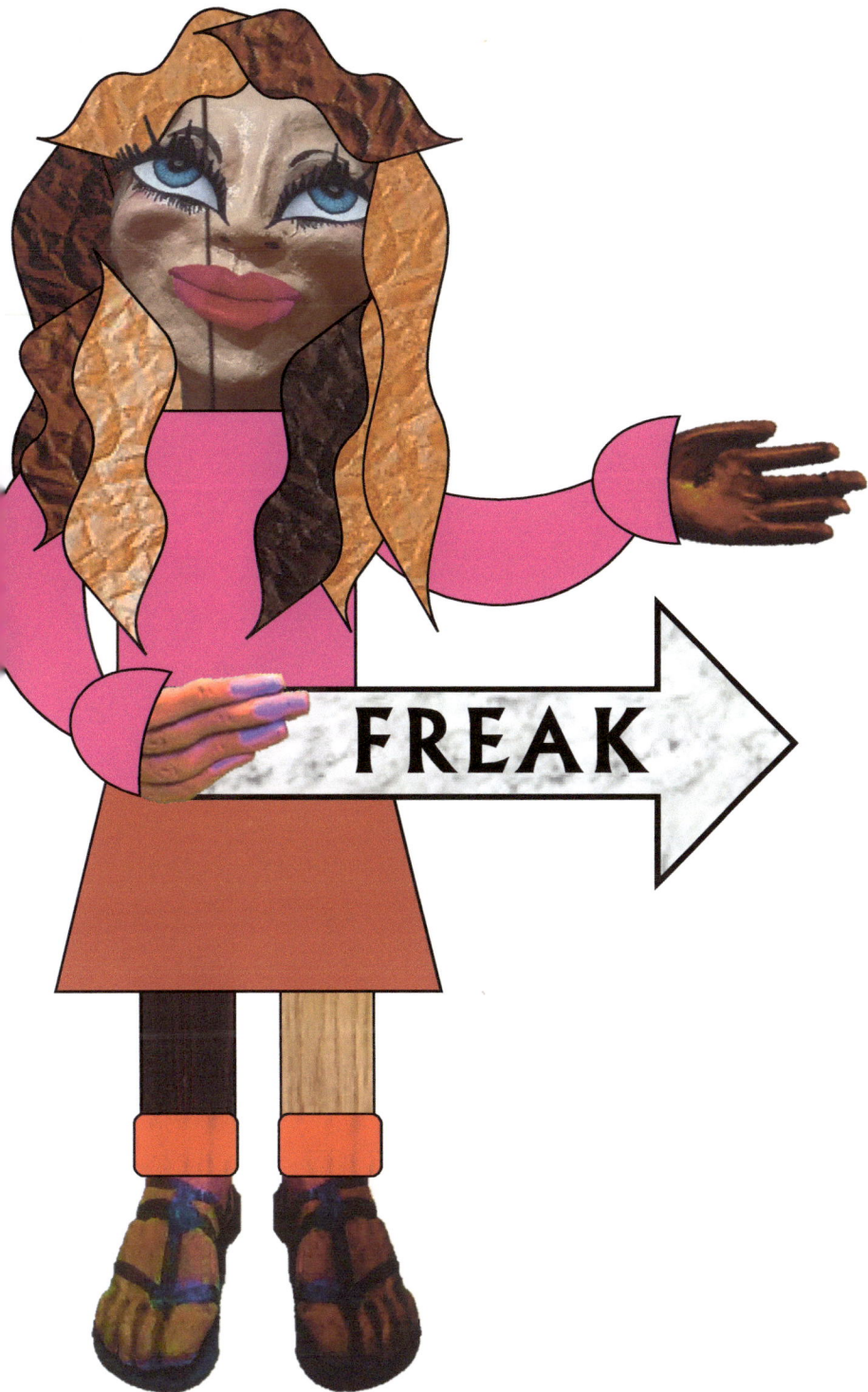

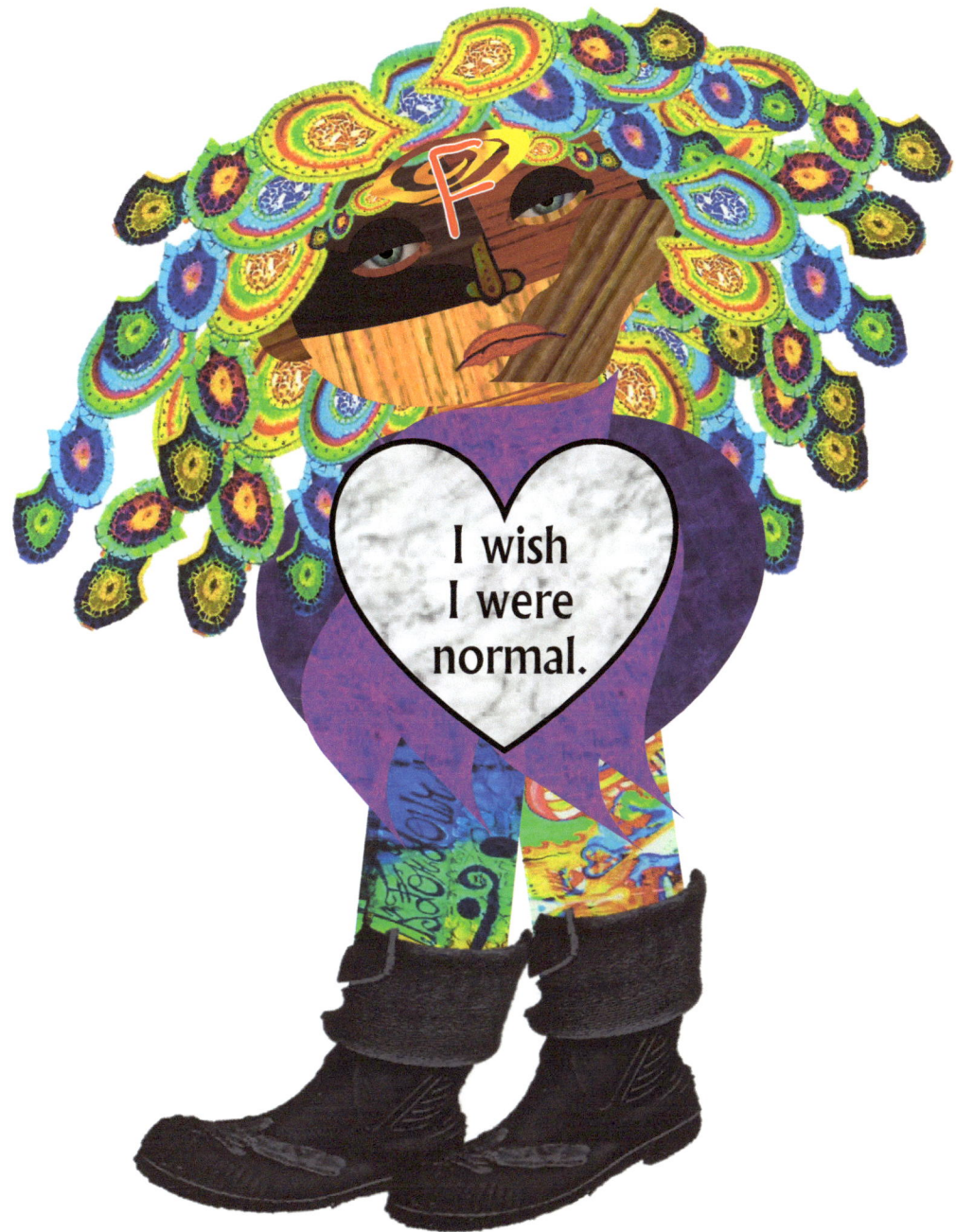

FREAK

I wish
I were
normal.

*Not* perfect in the sense that
our caves are comfortable,
or our feet accustomed to a life without fields,
or that our wounds warrant denial
instead of healing.

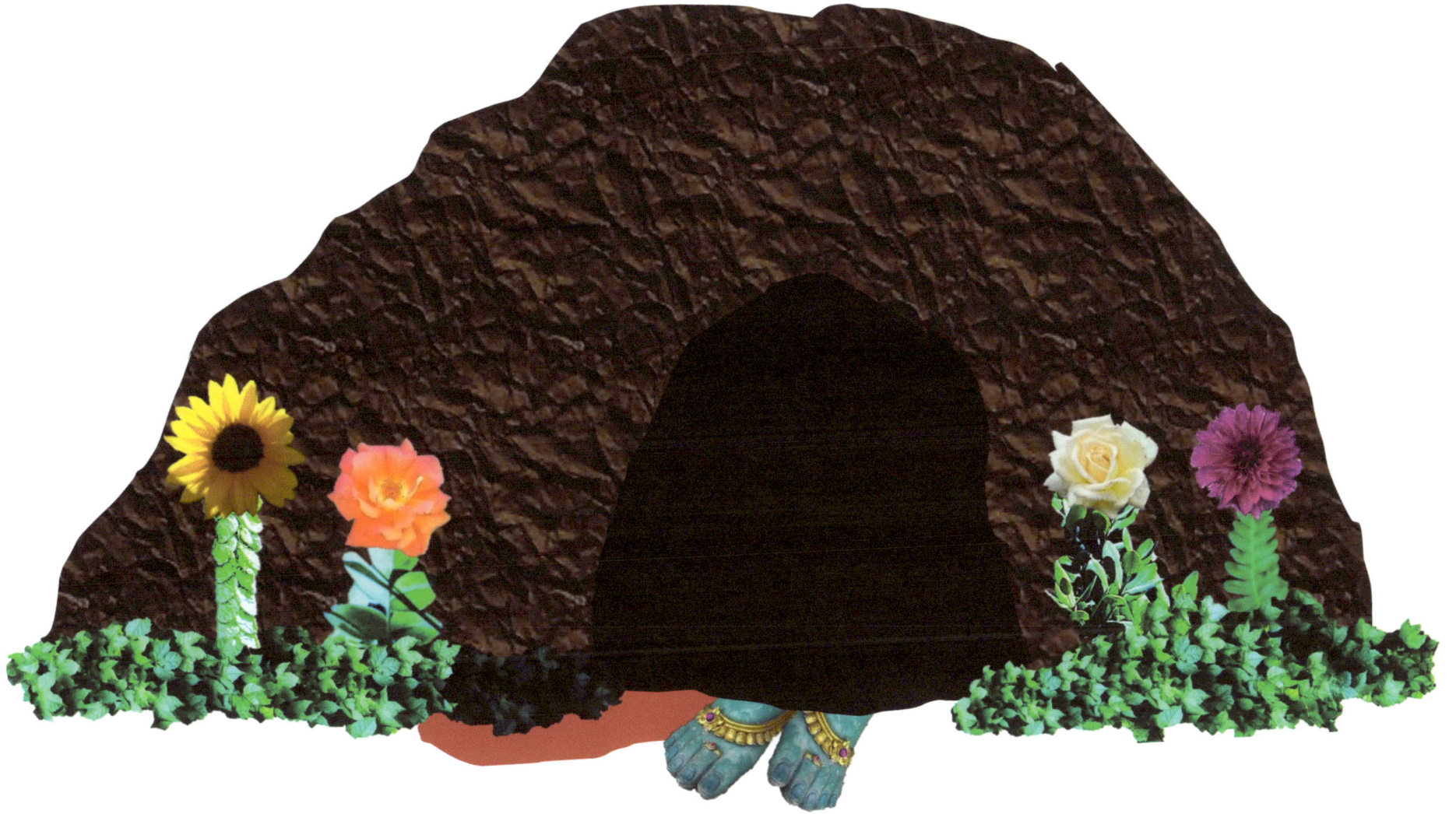

*Not* perfect in the sense that
suicidal thoughts
convincingly claim
that the grave is our only hope
for change.

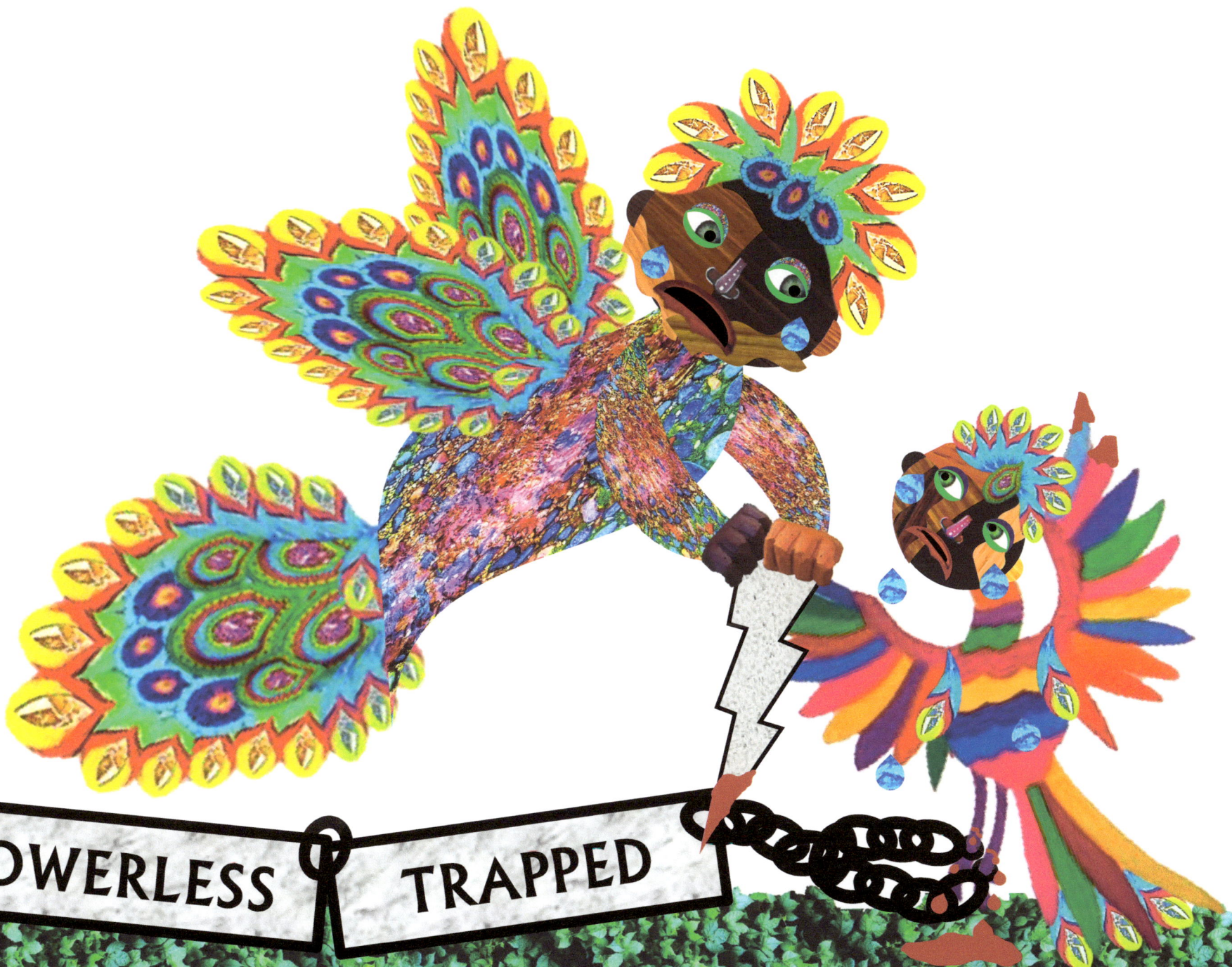

POWERLESS    TRAPPED

*Not* perfect in the sense that
our fallen sisters and brothers,
via far-too-early exits from this world,
imprinted deaths upon our hearts
that overshadowed their

# LIVES

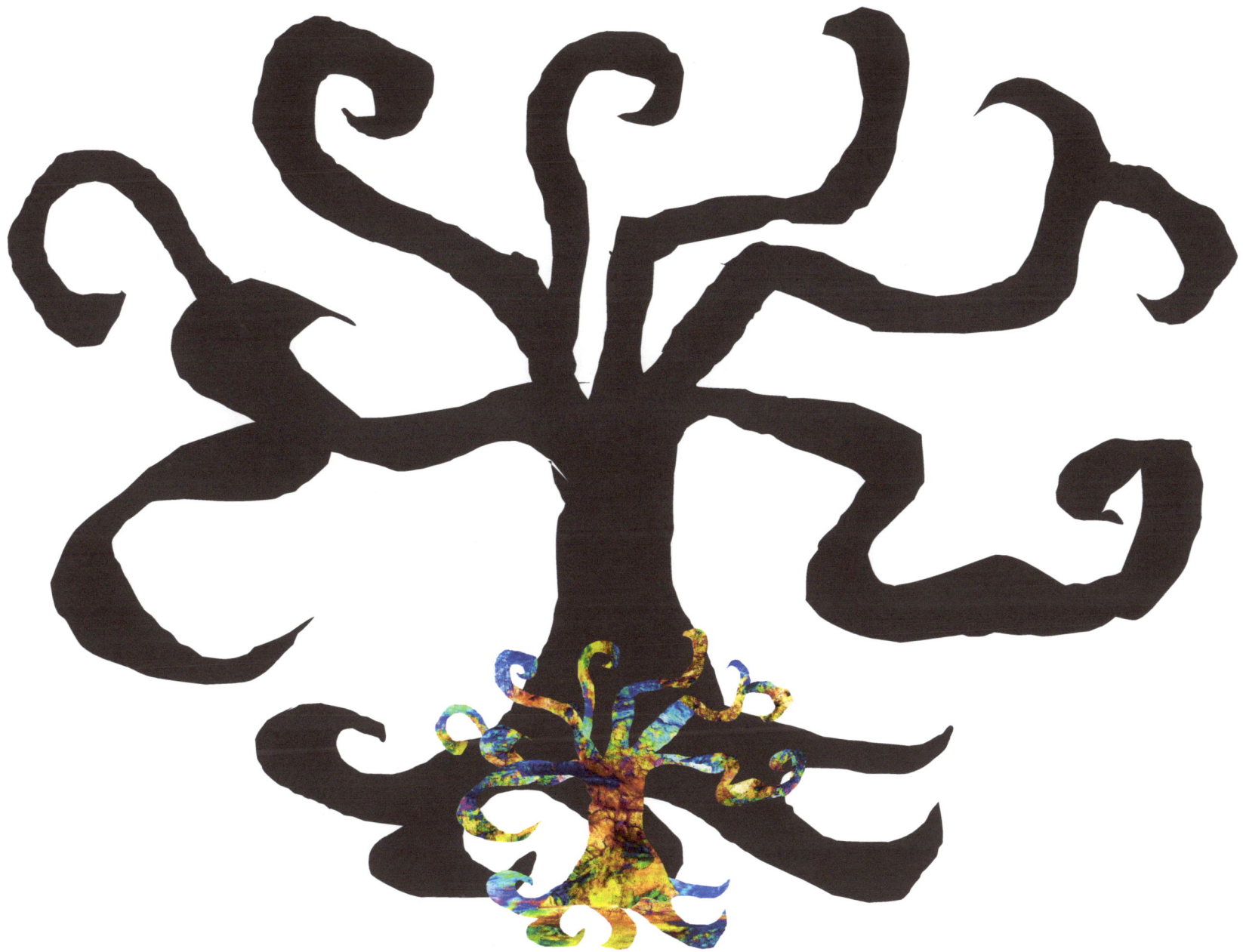

and all the

# LOVE

they gave
when they were here.

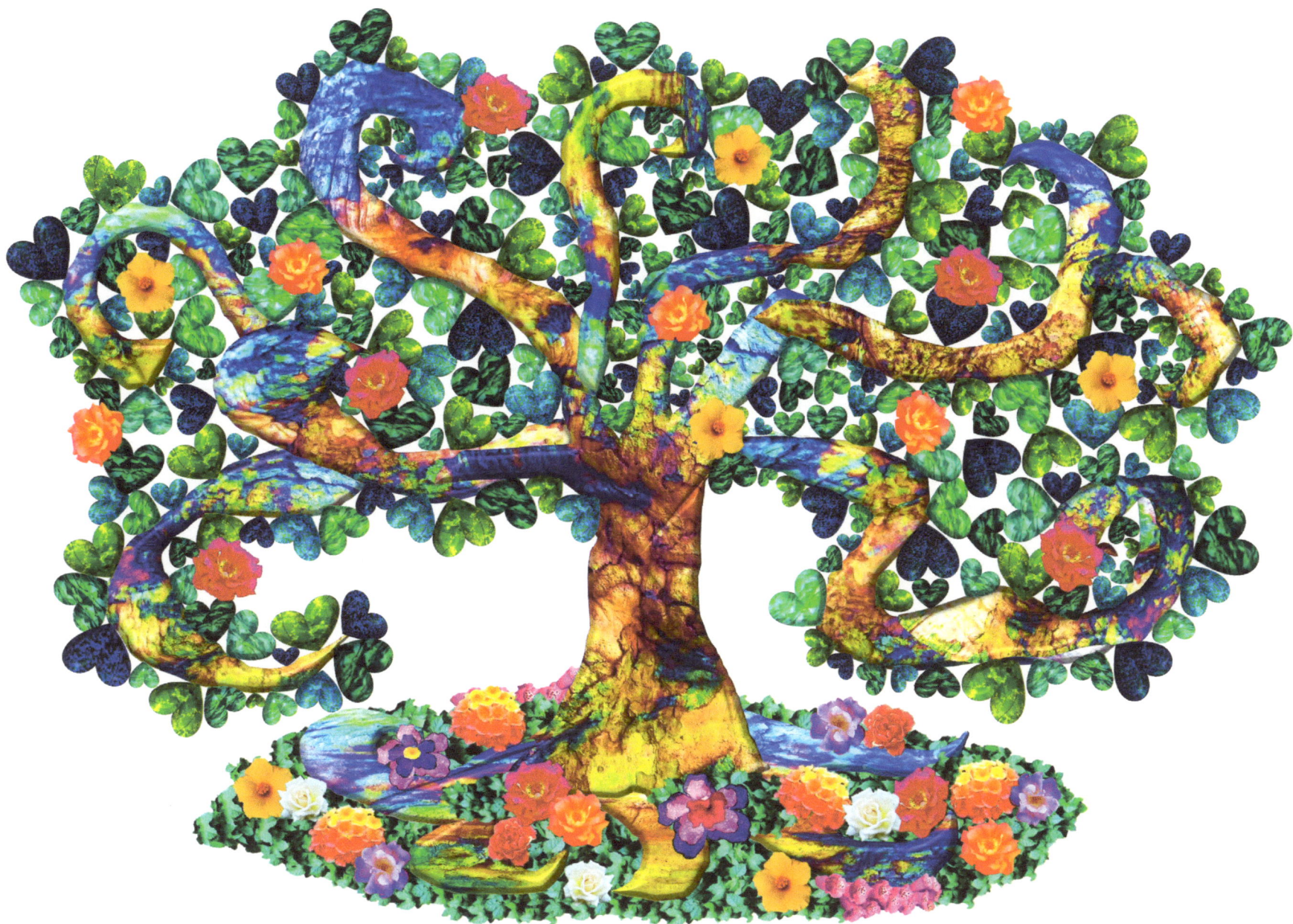

We are perfect in the sense that
the light inside us,
like the light inside you,
was sourced from the stars.

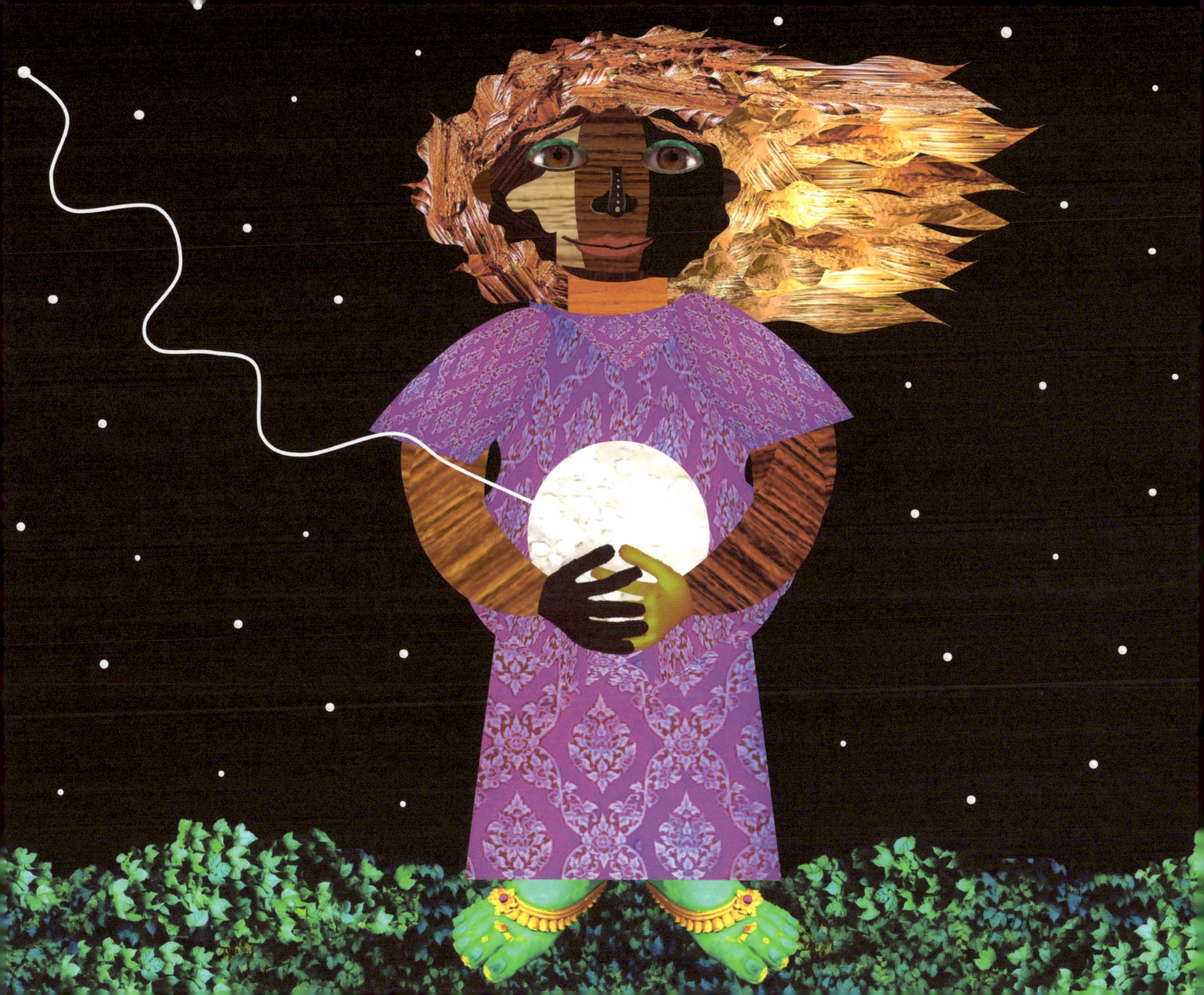

At our births,
just like at yours,
wonder beamed with pride and boasted,
"Look at the marvel that has just entered this world!"

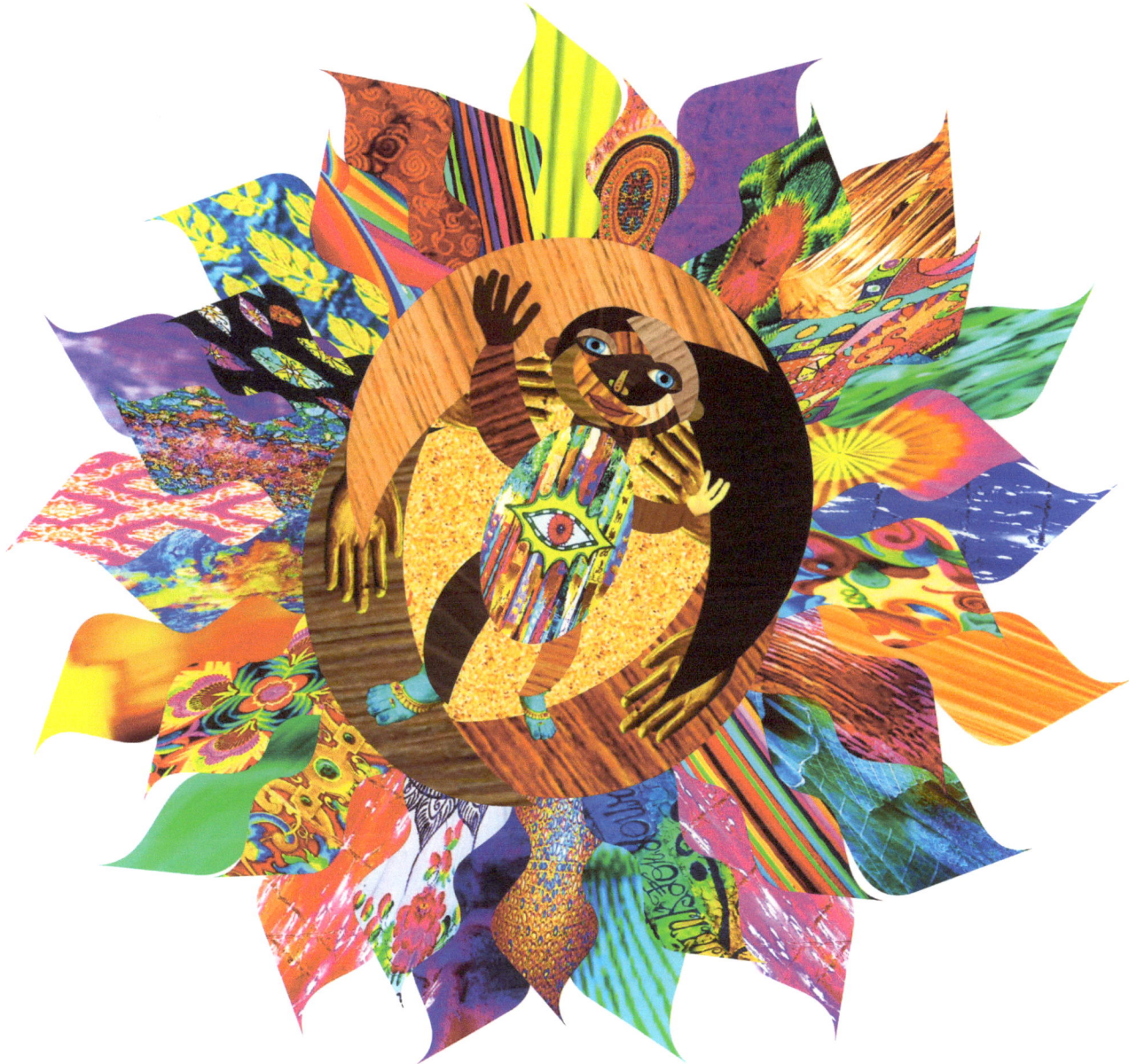

And at our deaths,
whenever and however they come to us,
wonder will salute its exquisite creation.

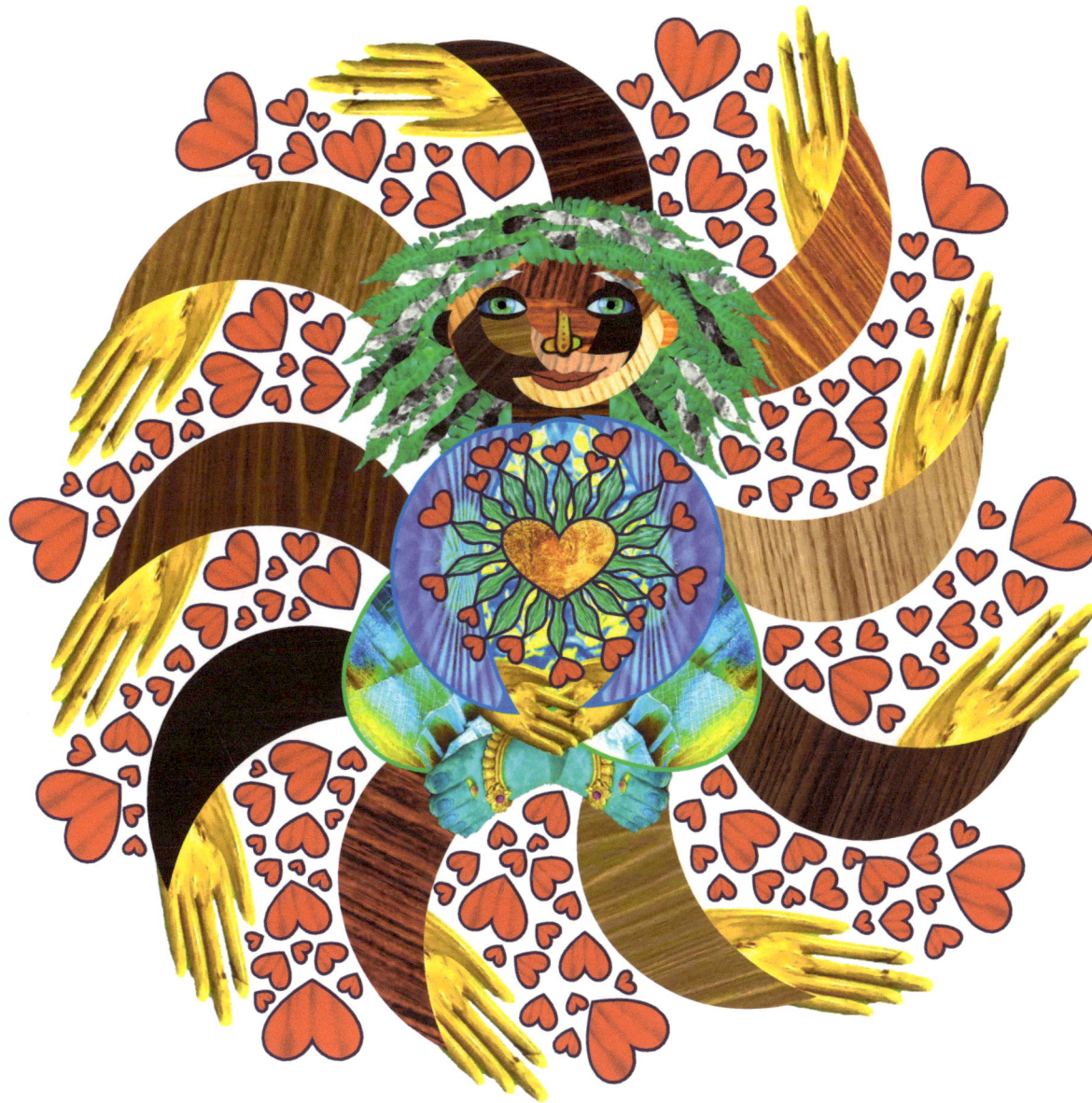

We are perfect in the sense that
the Grand Composers
prepare spaces for our notes by night
and clutch hope to their hearts by day
that we will fulfill the need of music
to birth new songs
and pen the divine melodies that
only we can write.

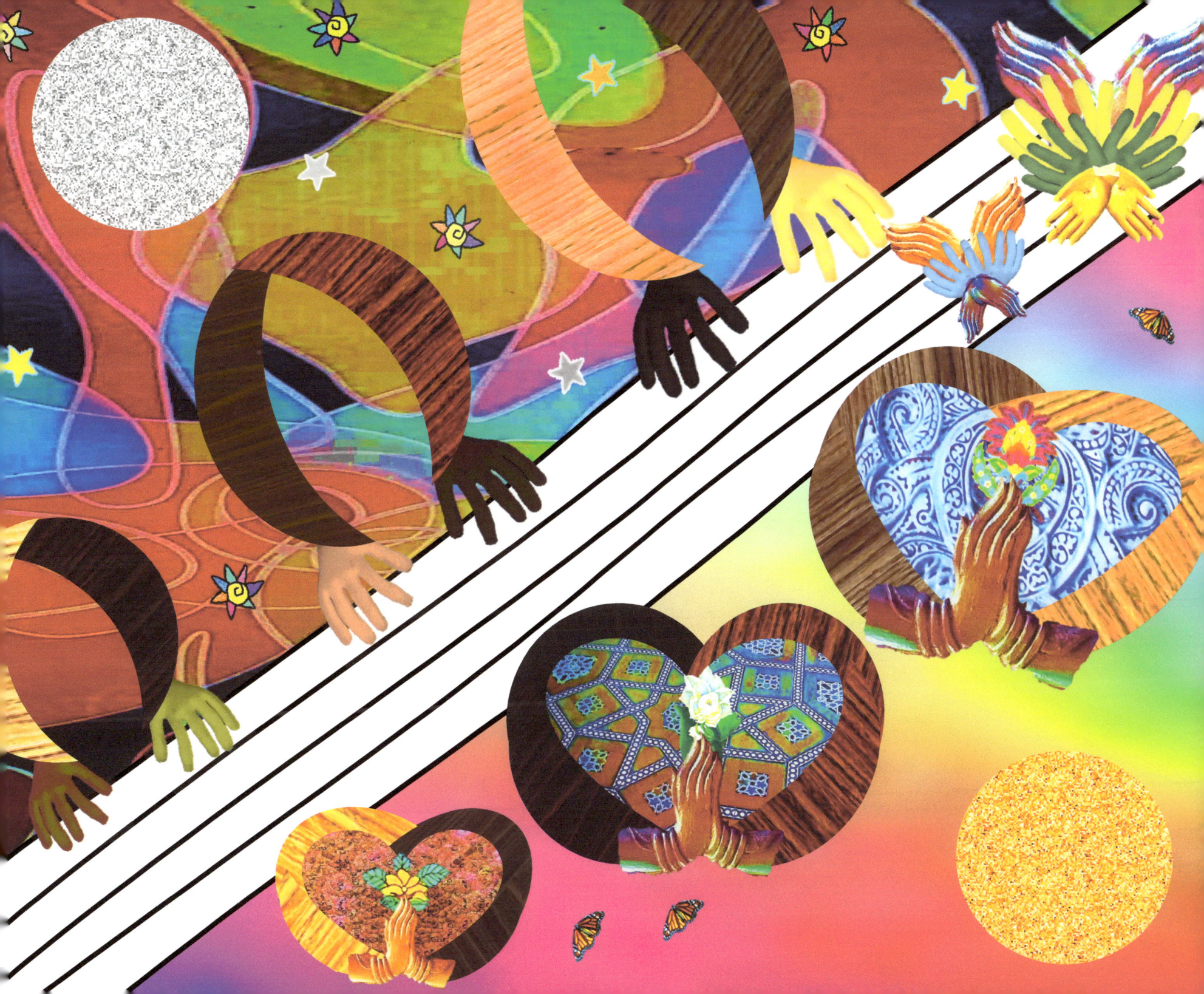

We are perfect in the sense that
love *always* looks us square in the soul
and shouts with all its strength
so it will be heard and believed
above the brutal din:

"Do *not* mistake lies for truths.
*YOU* are the reason I rise."

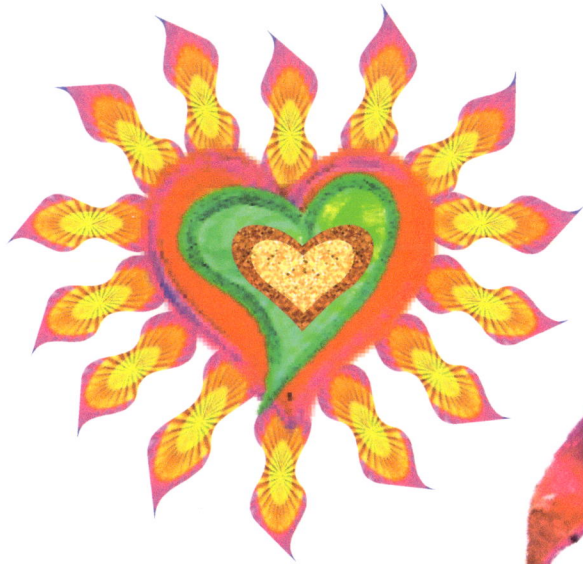

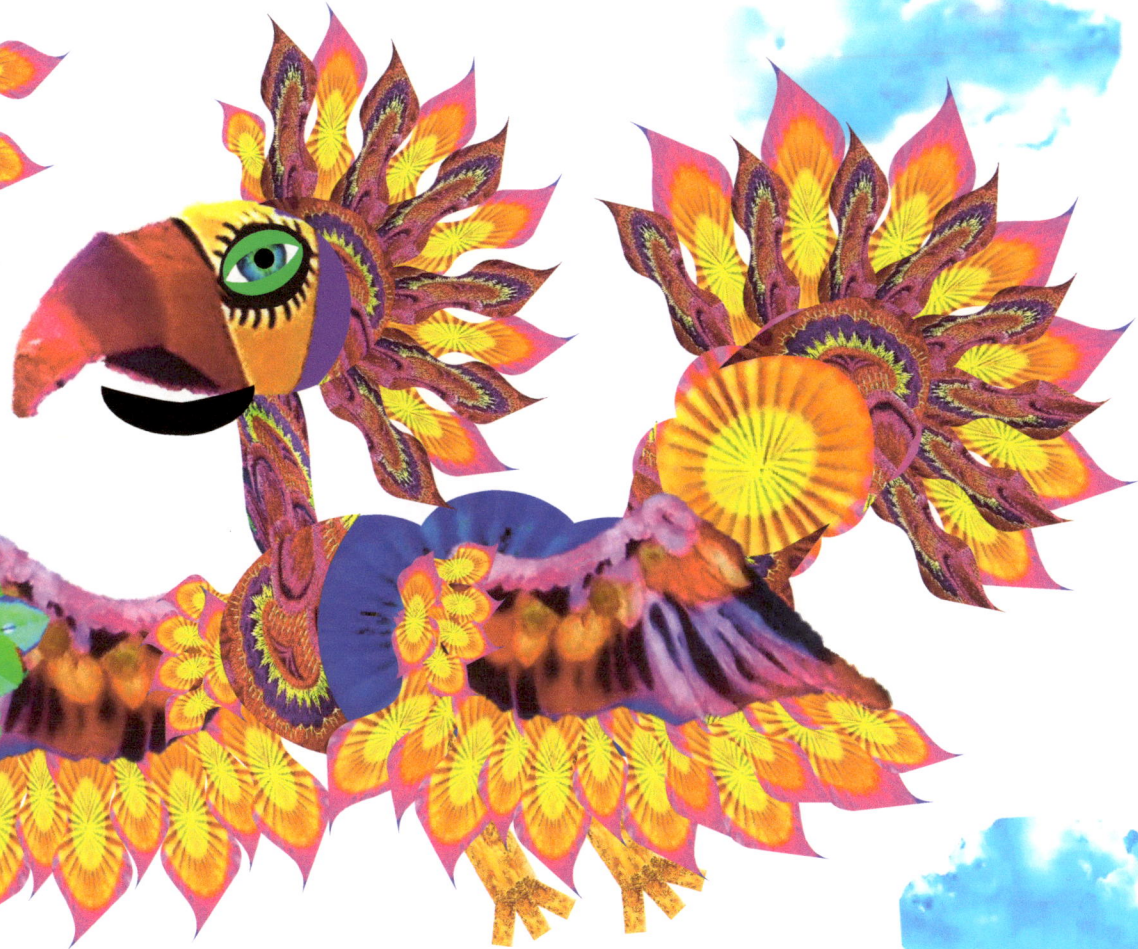

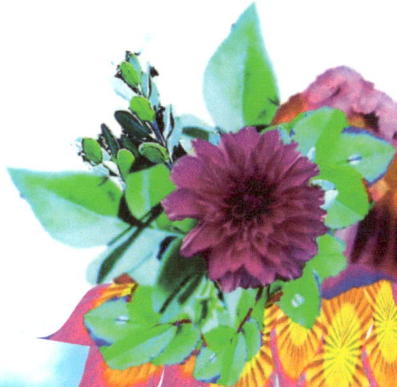

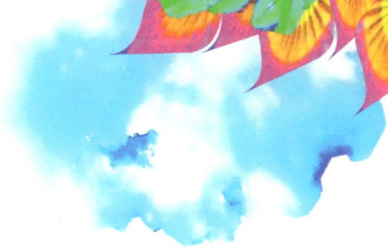

The new normal.
It can be a revolution
instead of a repetition.

If the new normal can be anything,
let it be this:

As we stand before each other,
even on our darkest days,
we will lower our heads,
clasp our hands in a sign of the prayers
that we have the power to answer, and say,

"The light in me bows to the light in you."

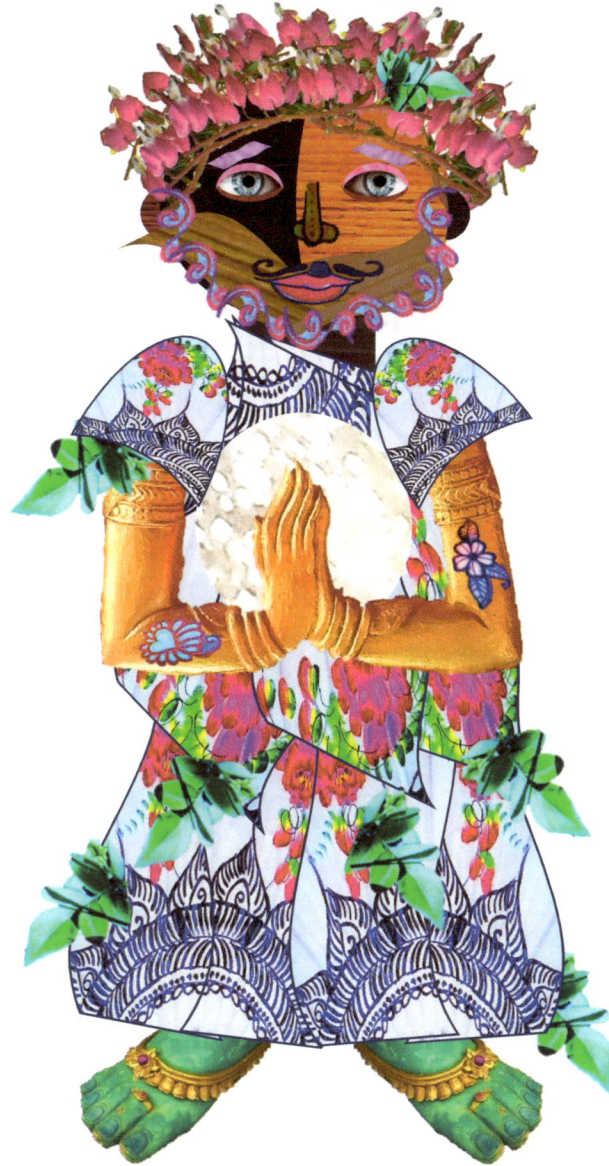

The question

"How do you feel?"

will always
be asked with sincerity
and answered with honesty.

Comprehension
will not be a prerequisite for
compassion.

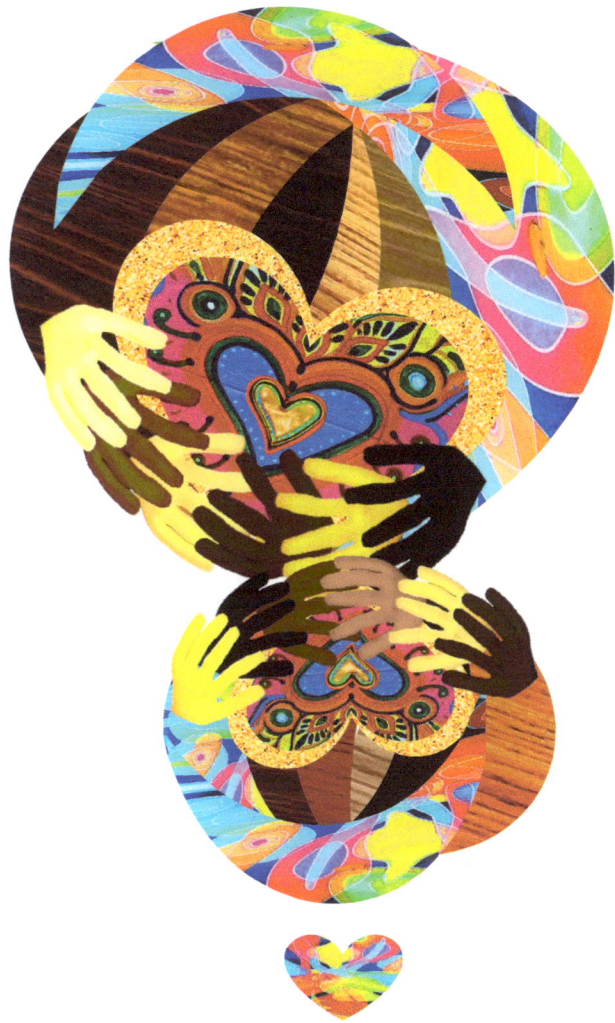

The question

"Why should I go on?"

will never be asked,
for every breath out and every breath in
will offer and return the same reality:

You are loved.
You are needed.
You are not alone.

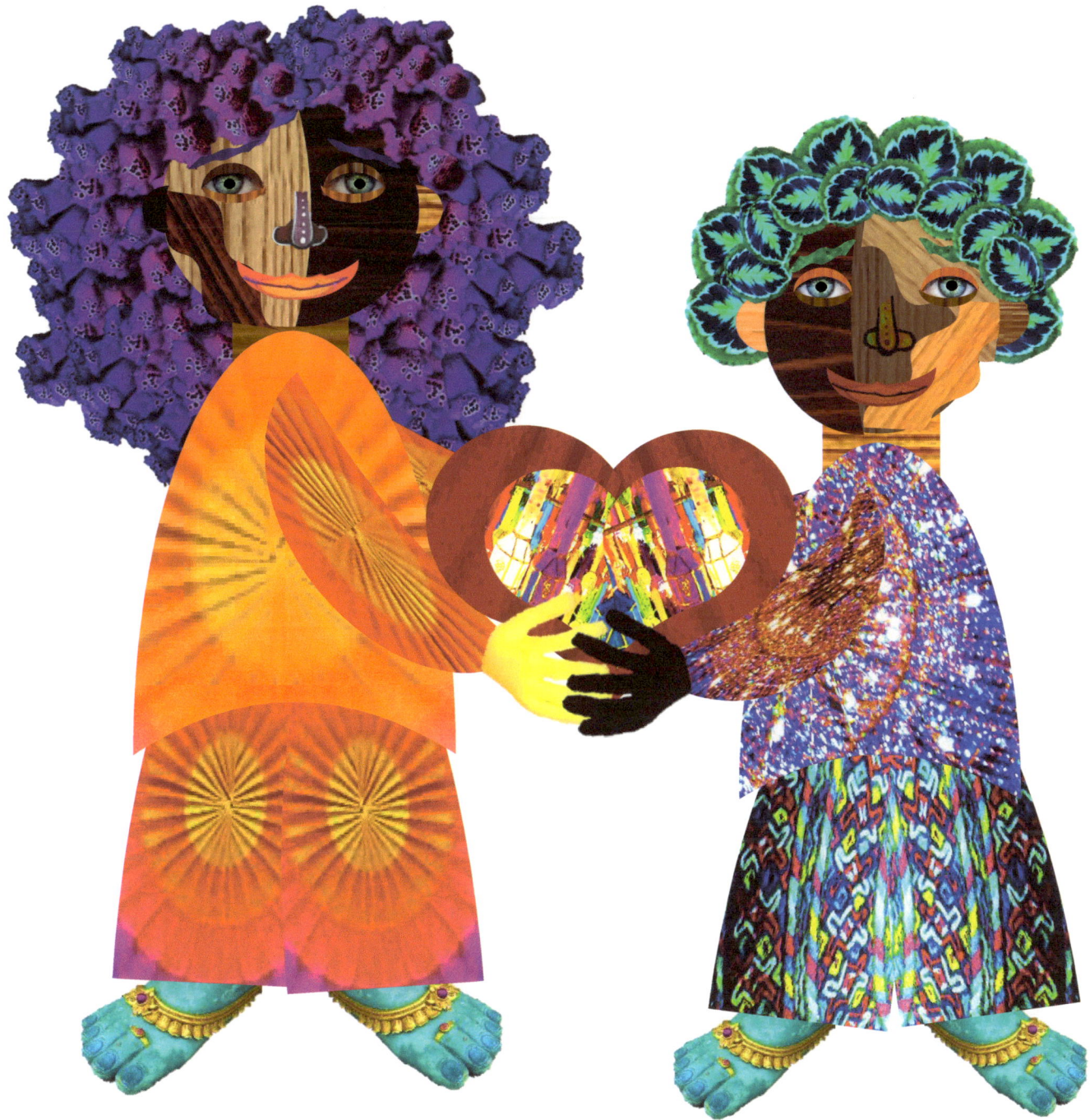

To feel deeply will be a mark of strength.

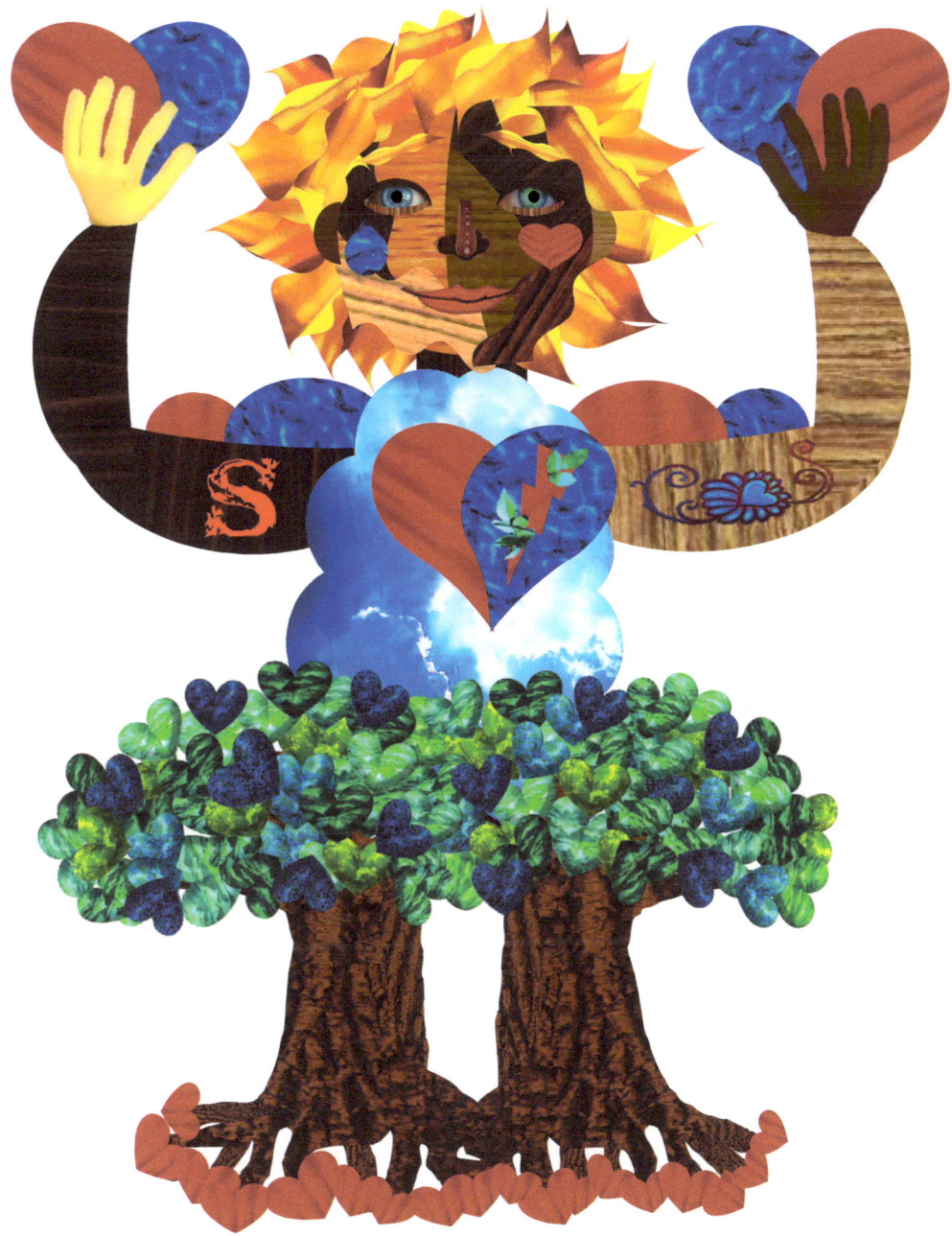

To weep openly will be met
with an embrace from the rain, who cries,
"At long last you understand!"

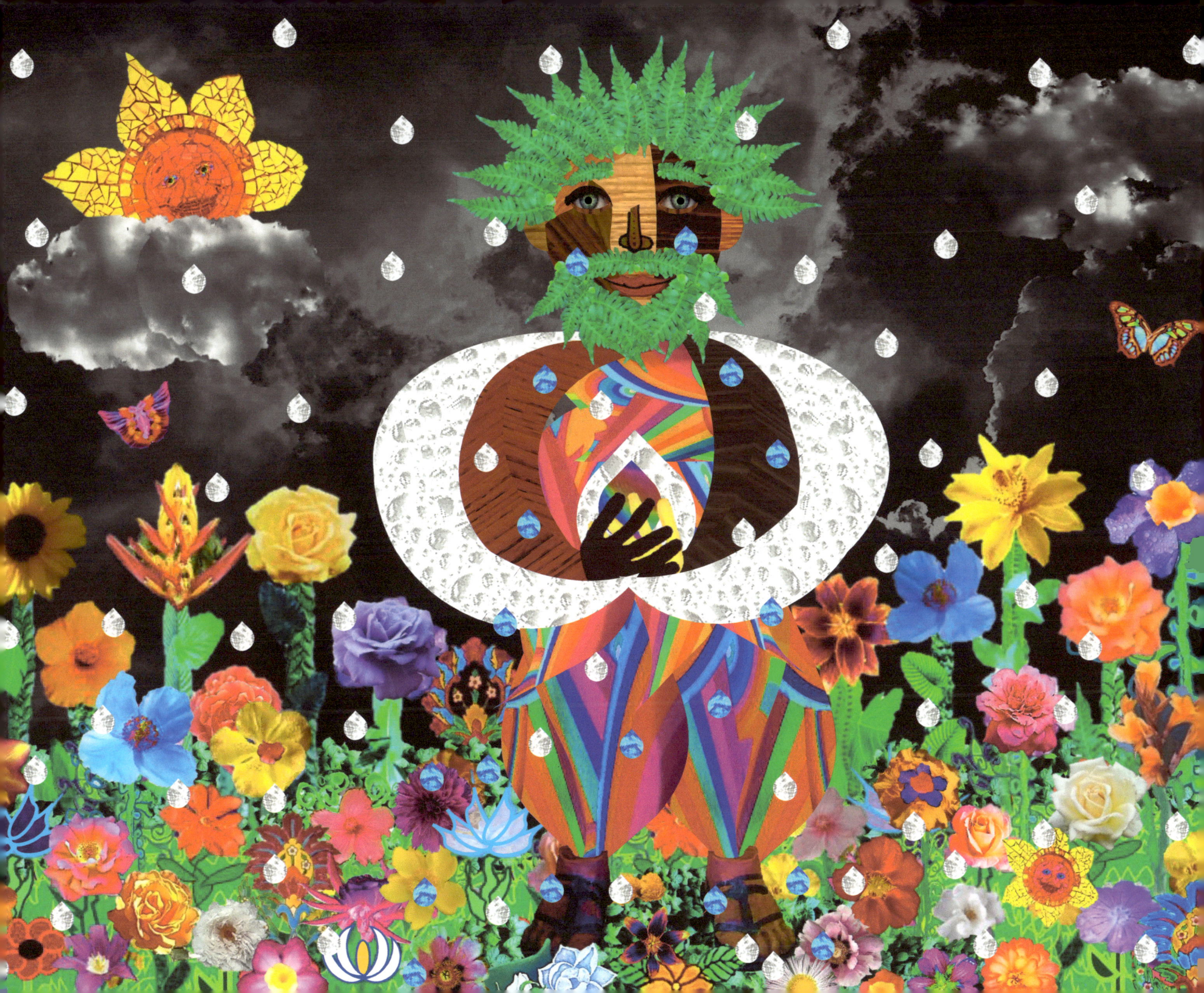

To laugh loudly will be as common as kindness.

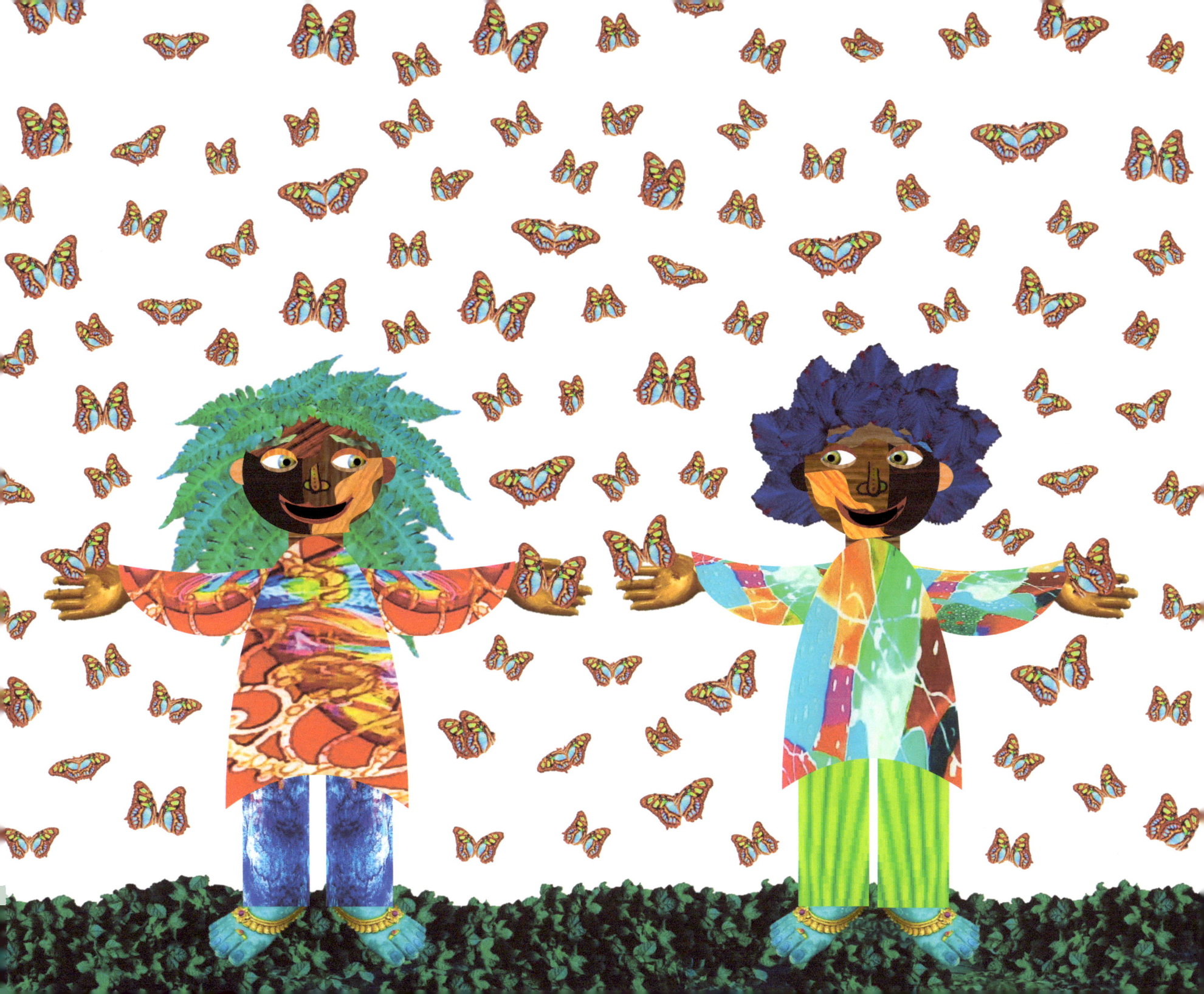

The paths we walk will be soft and wide.
They will be laid with magic,
and the signposts will read
*BELIEVE*.

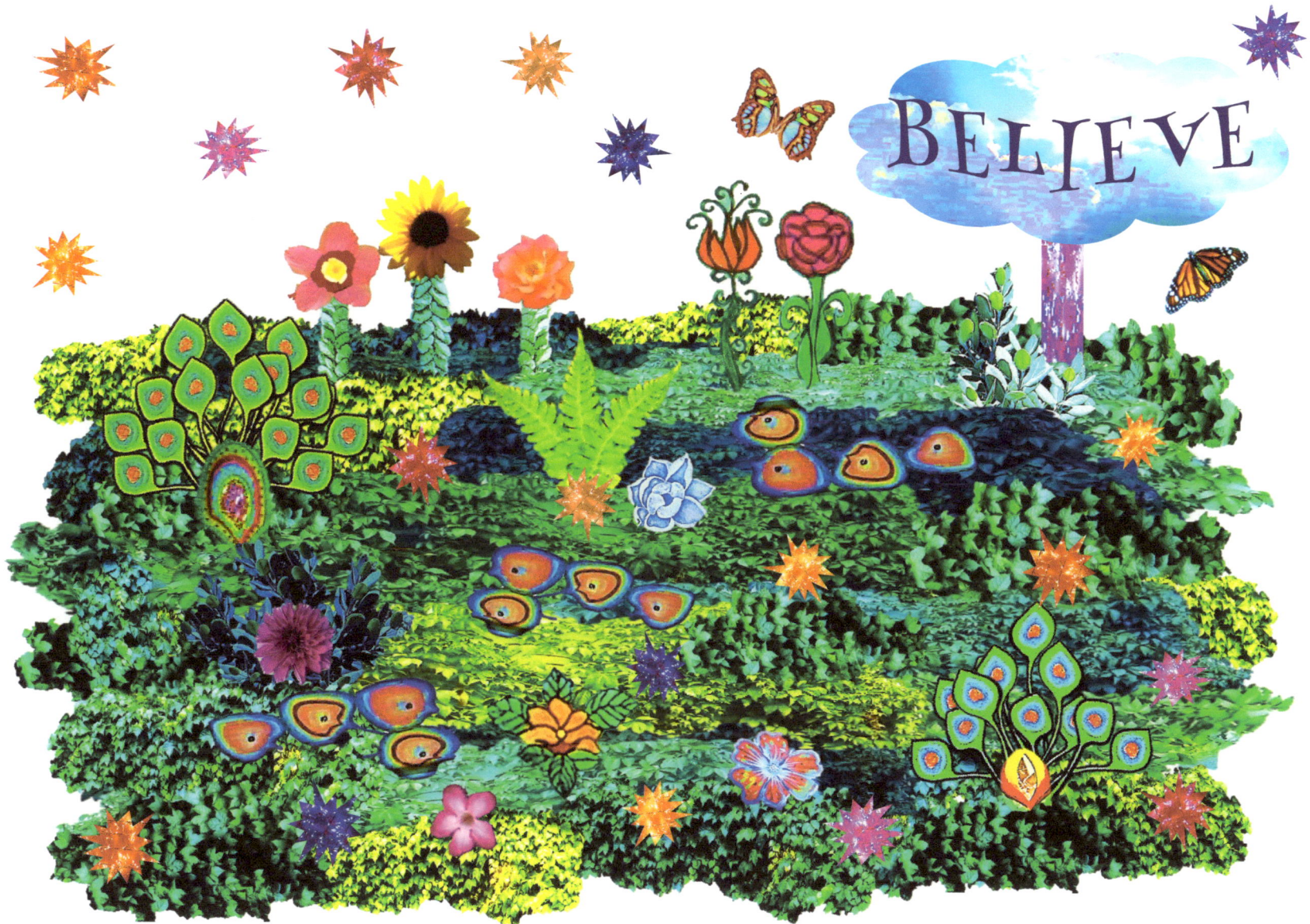

BELIEVE

Our steps will be slow
for our purpose will be clear:

Listen and sing.

Listen
until
the rose no longer need ask us
to pause in awe,
for her urgency and wisdom
will dwell in our bones.

ONE LIFE

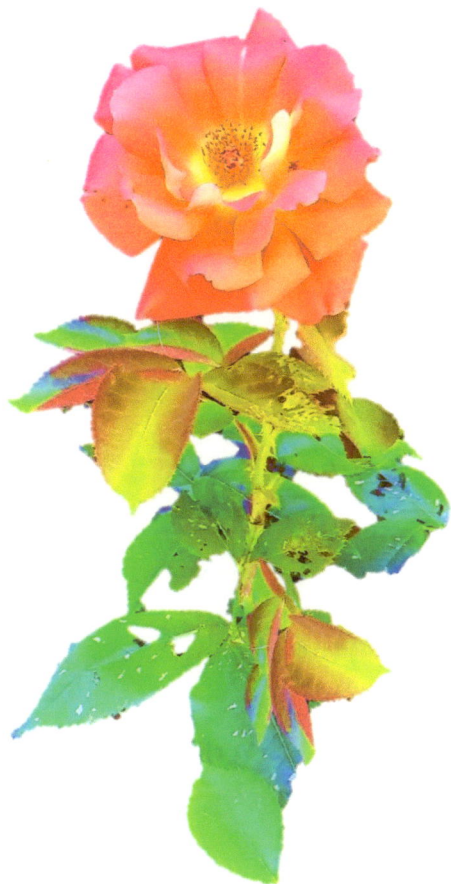

Listen
until
no child need ever beg to be heard,
for their voices will be our compass.

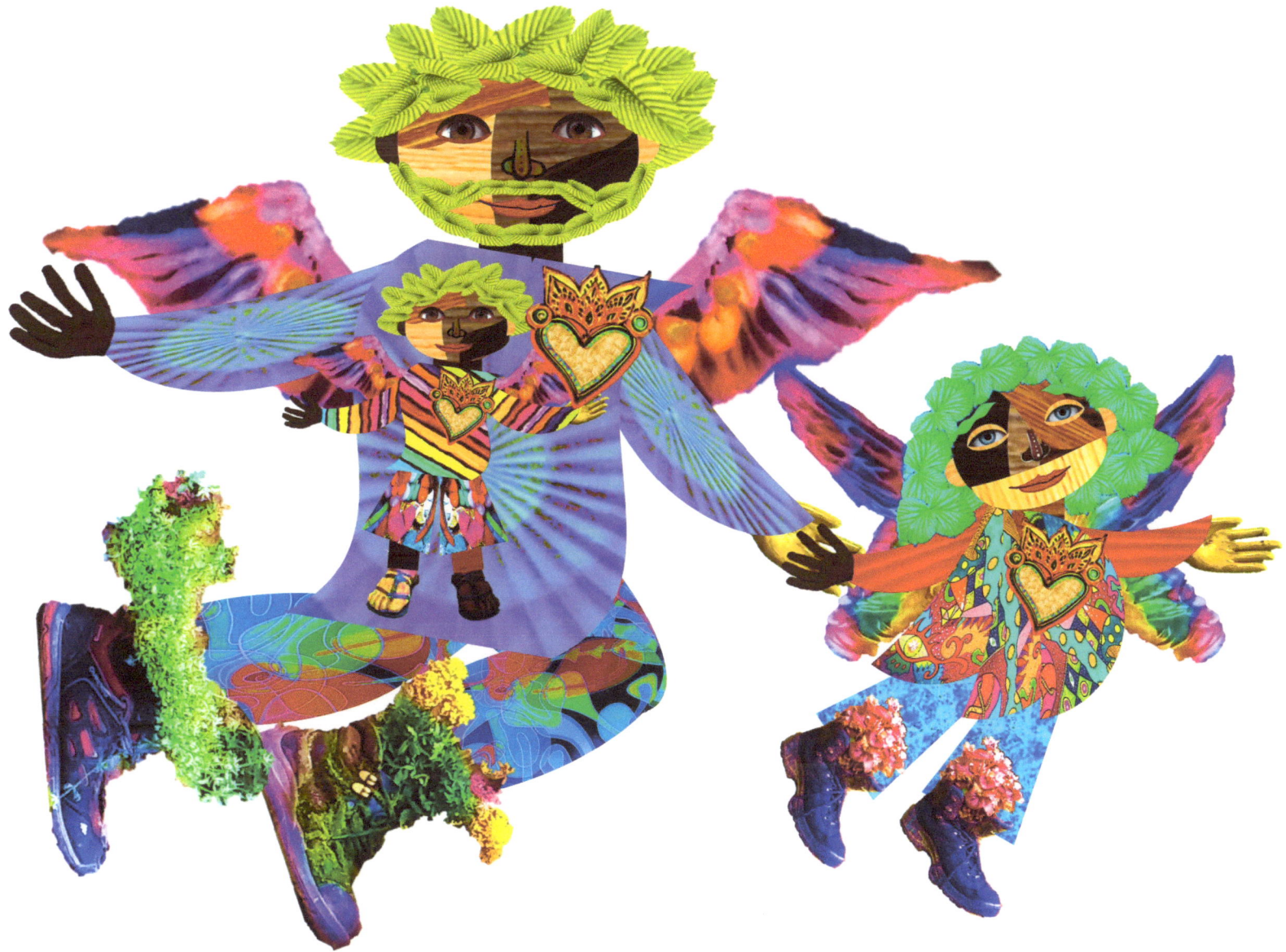

Sing
odes to joy and songs of love
with notes gathered from
the birthplace of beauty,
the origin of existence:
difference.

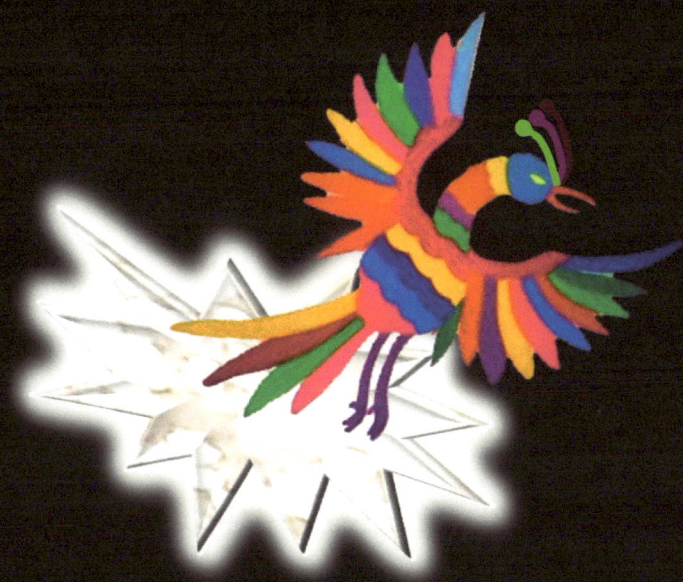

Sing
psalms of freedom
so peace will reign within and without;
so power will be the guardian of justice;
so no being will ever know shackles;
so no battle to be oneself need ever be fought.

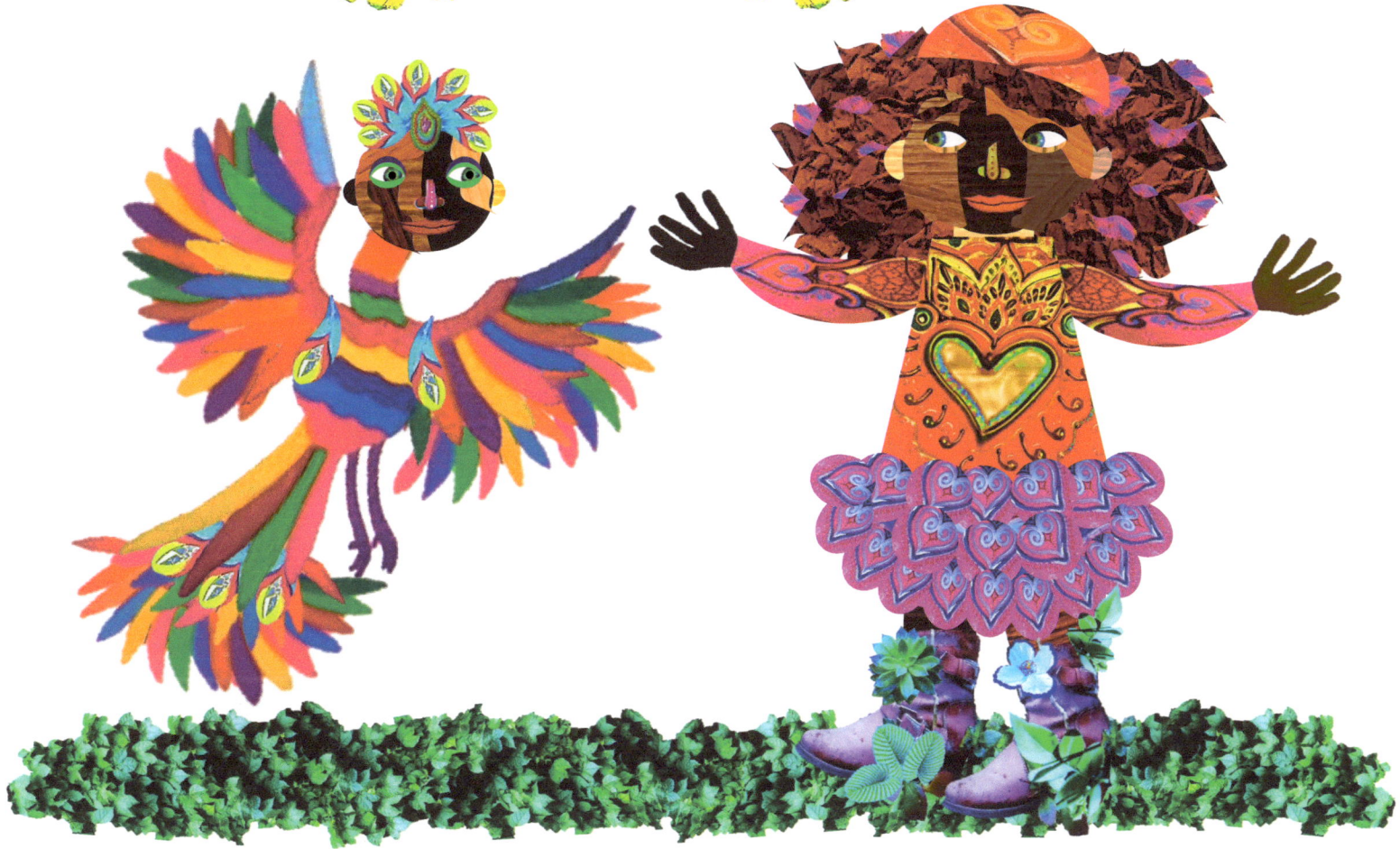
Freedom

Our meals will nourish body and soul,
for we will break bread side by side
in sacred circles upon the ground,
and at round tables that
equality has built and respect has set.
Every place will be marked
*Guest of Honor.*

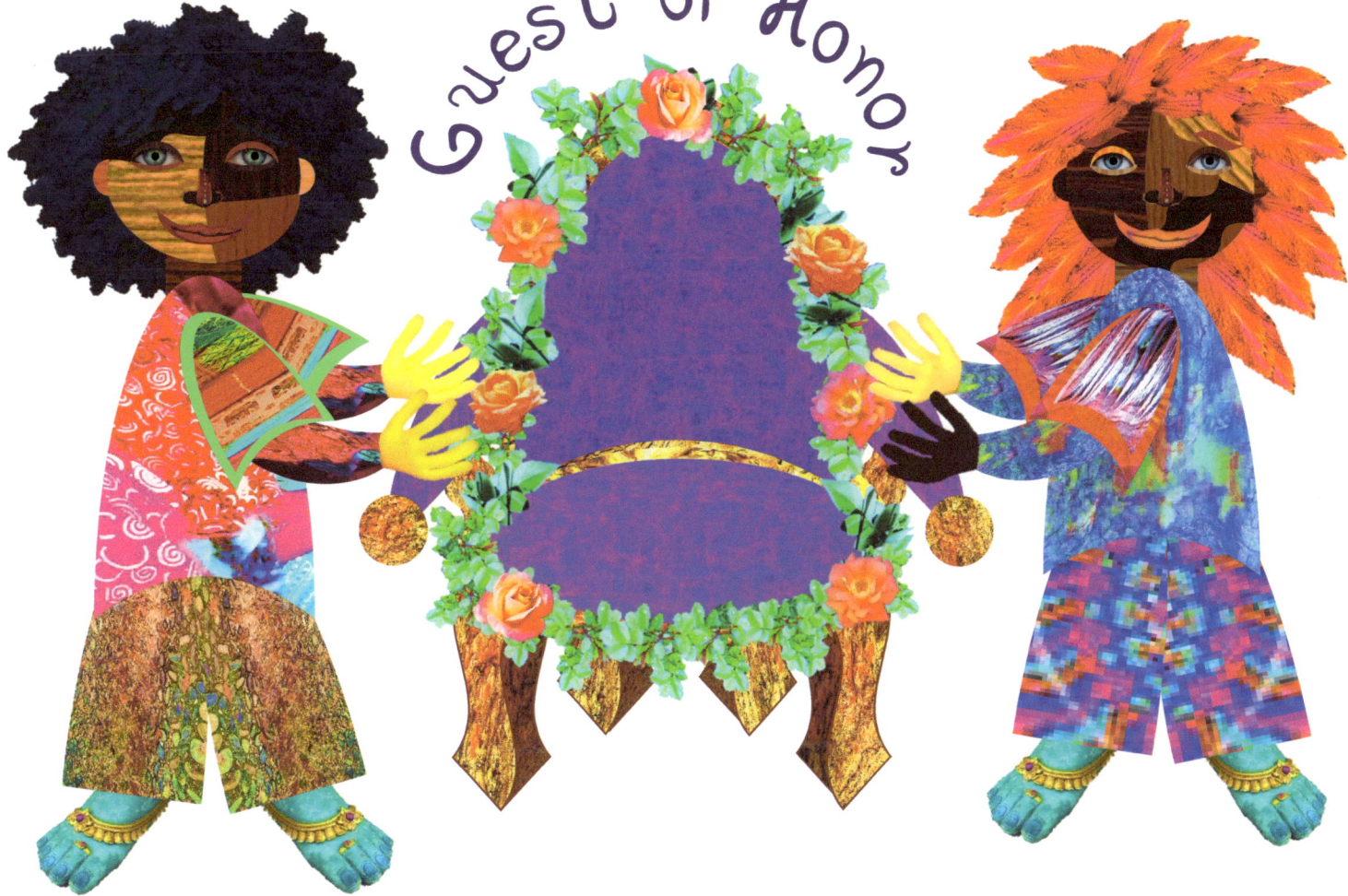

Guest of Honor

Strangers will trade in
loneliness for friendship
and
masks for truthfulness.

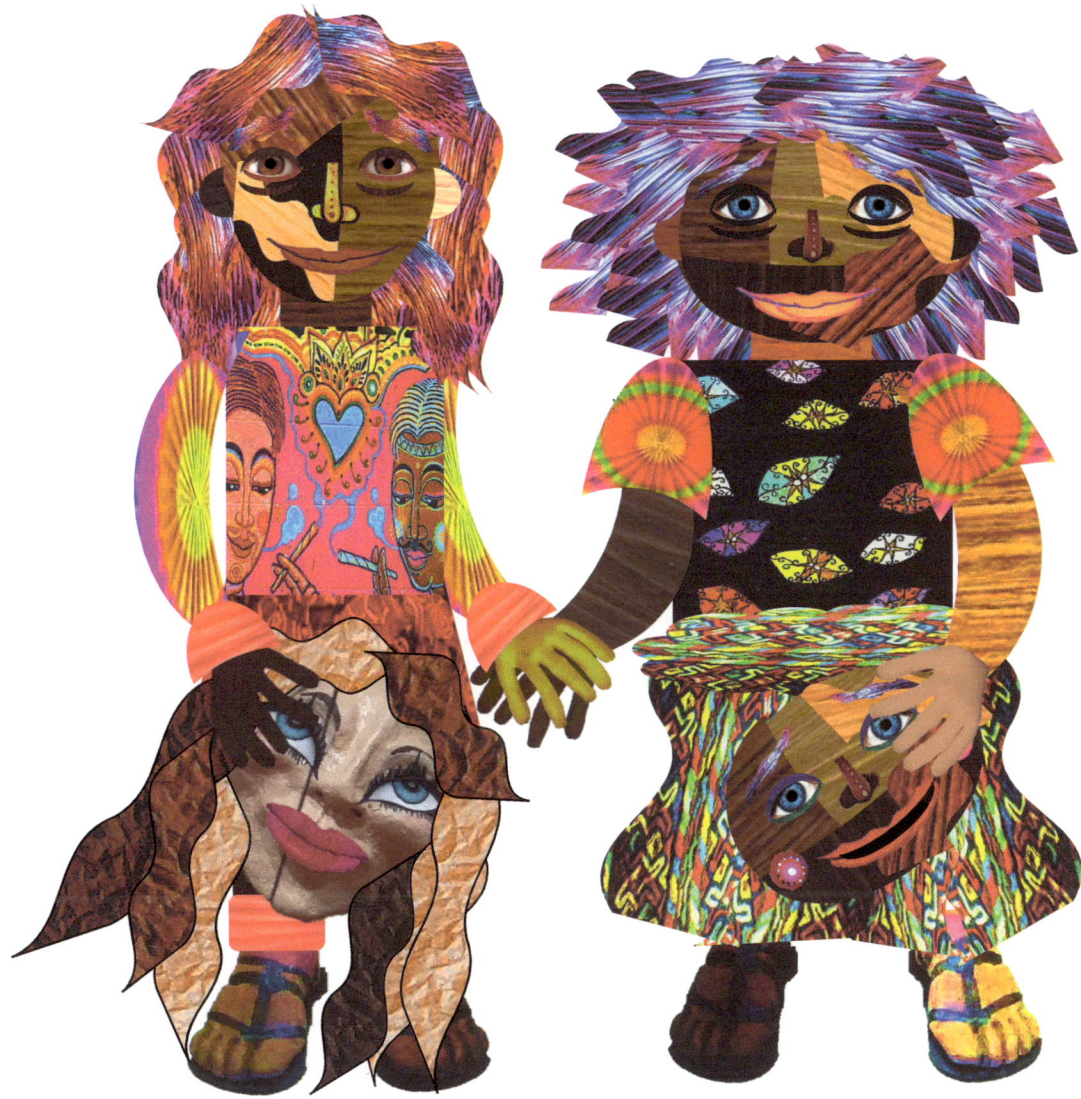

And fear will extol vulnerability, saying:
"You were not only brave—
you were right."

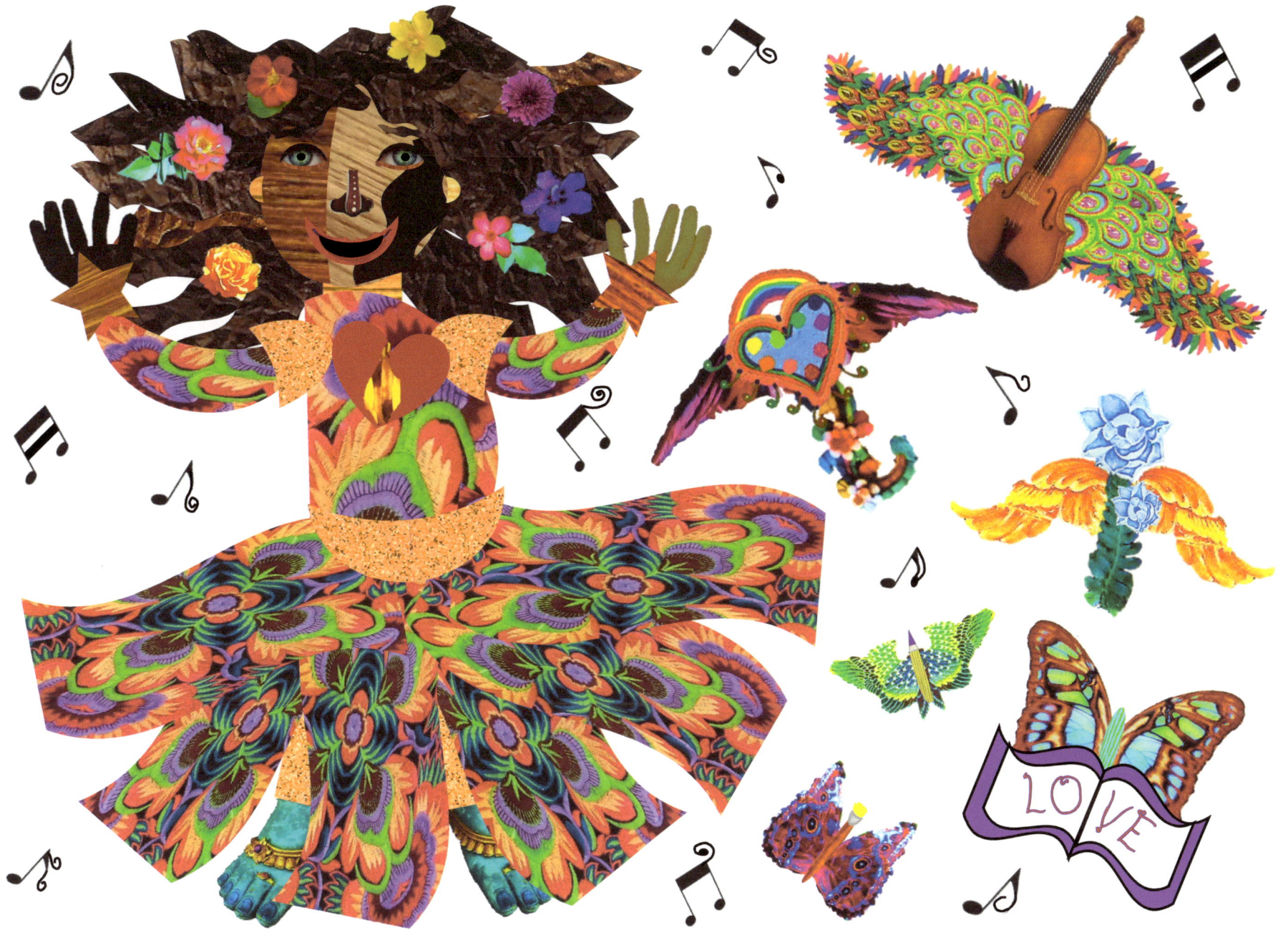

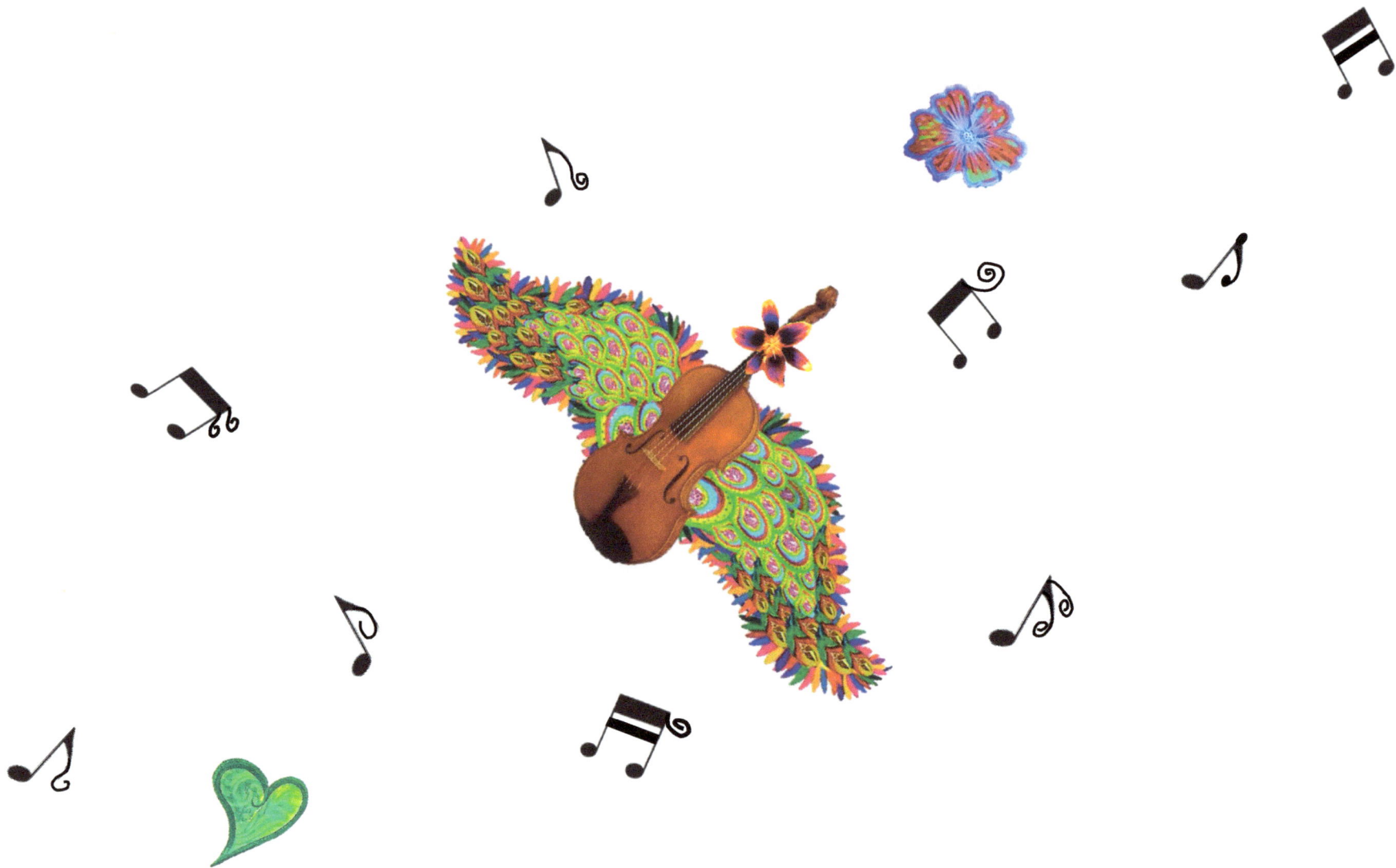

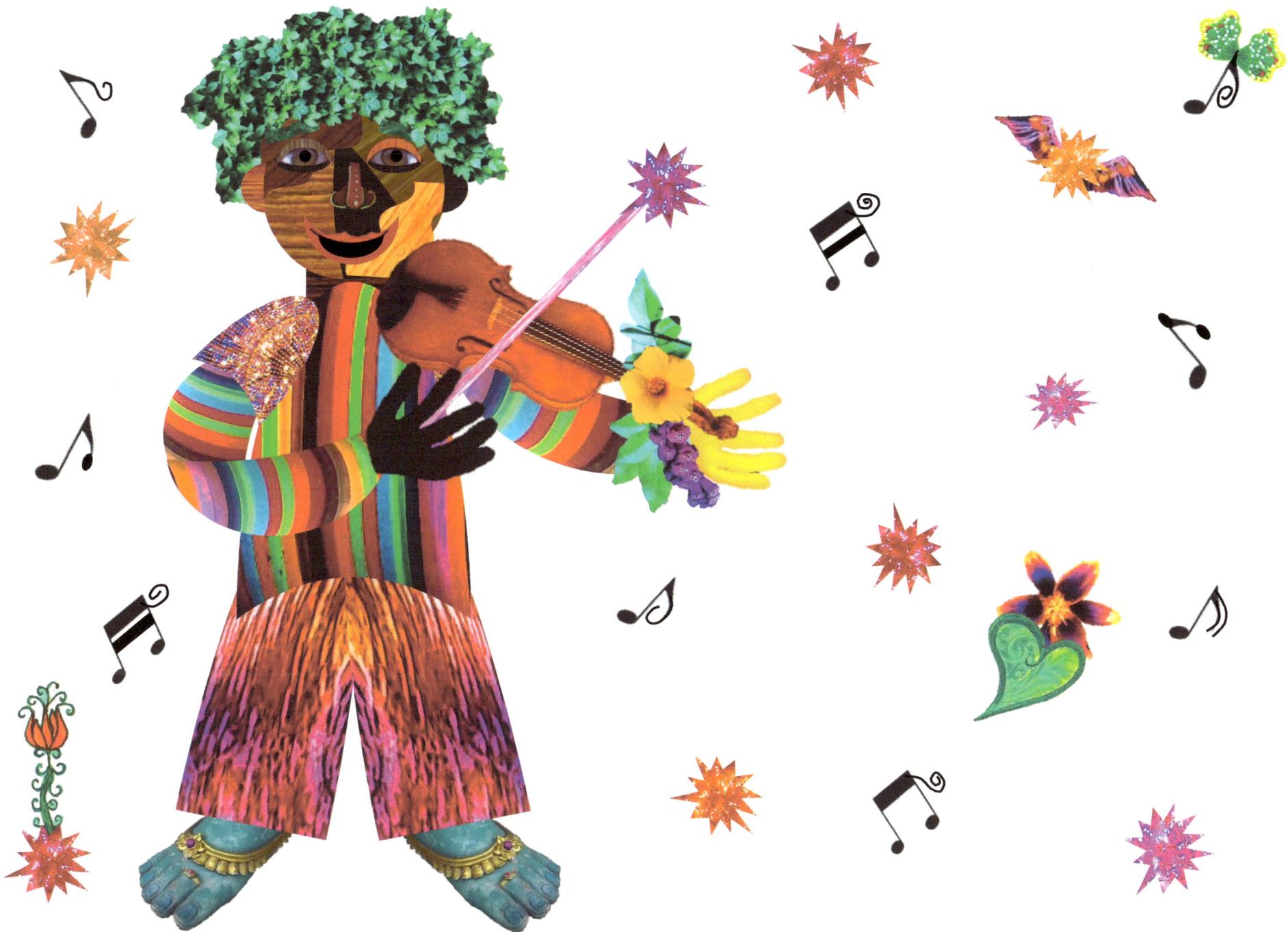

Sweet fruits will be eaten,
rivers respected,
insects and animals cherished,
and the earth will know
knees and hands and reverence
as we prostrate ourselves in gratitude
for her generosity.

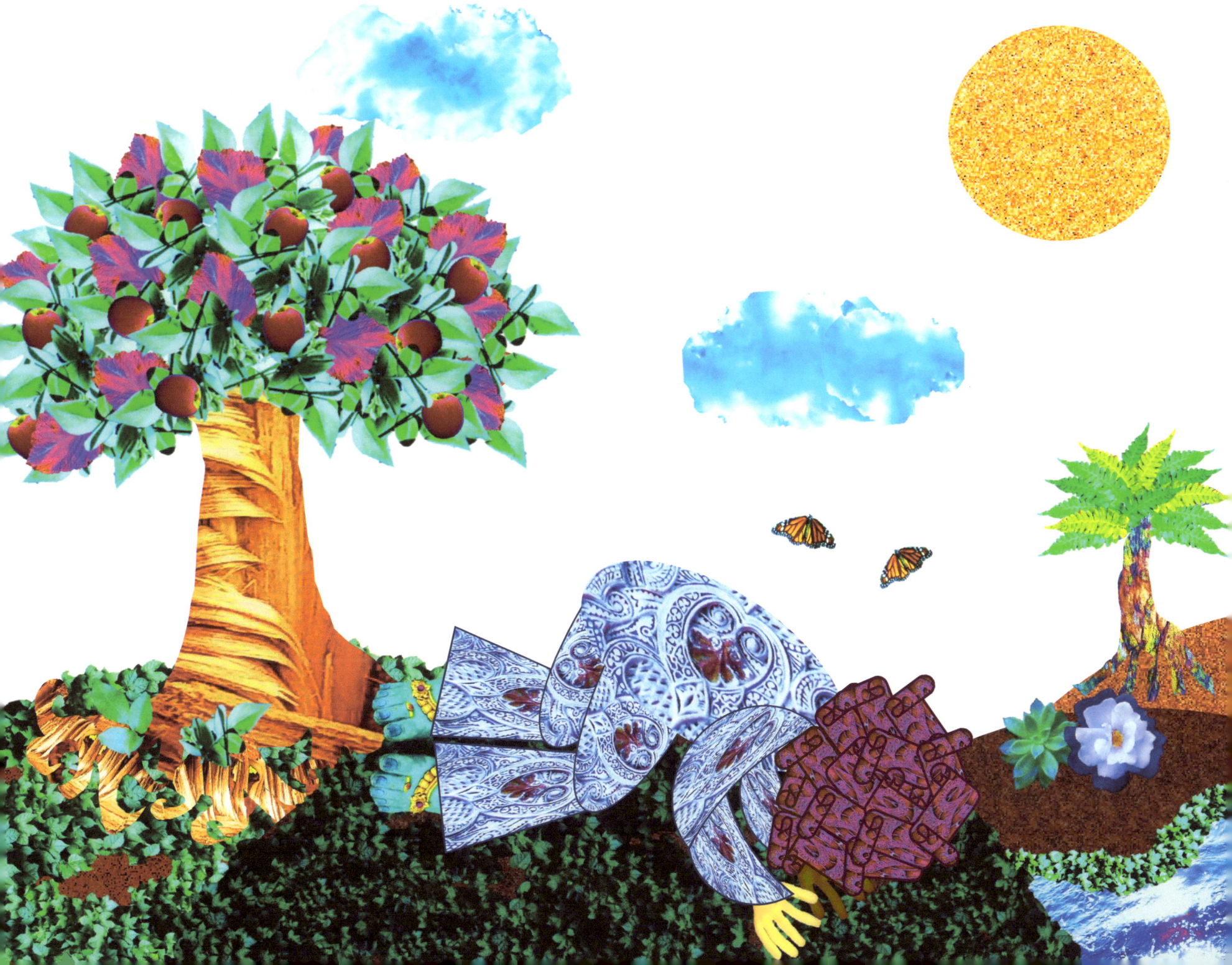

We will learn the planet's foremost teaching:
how to share instead of own.

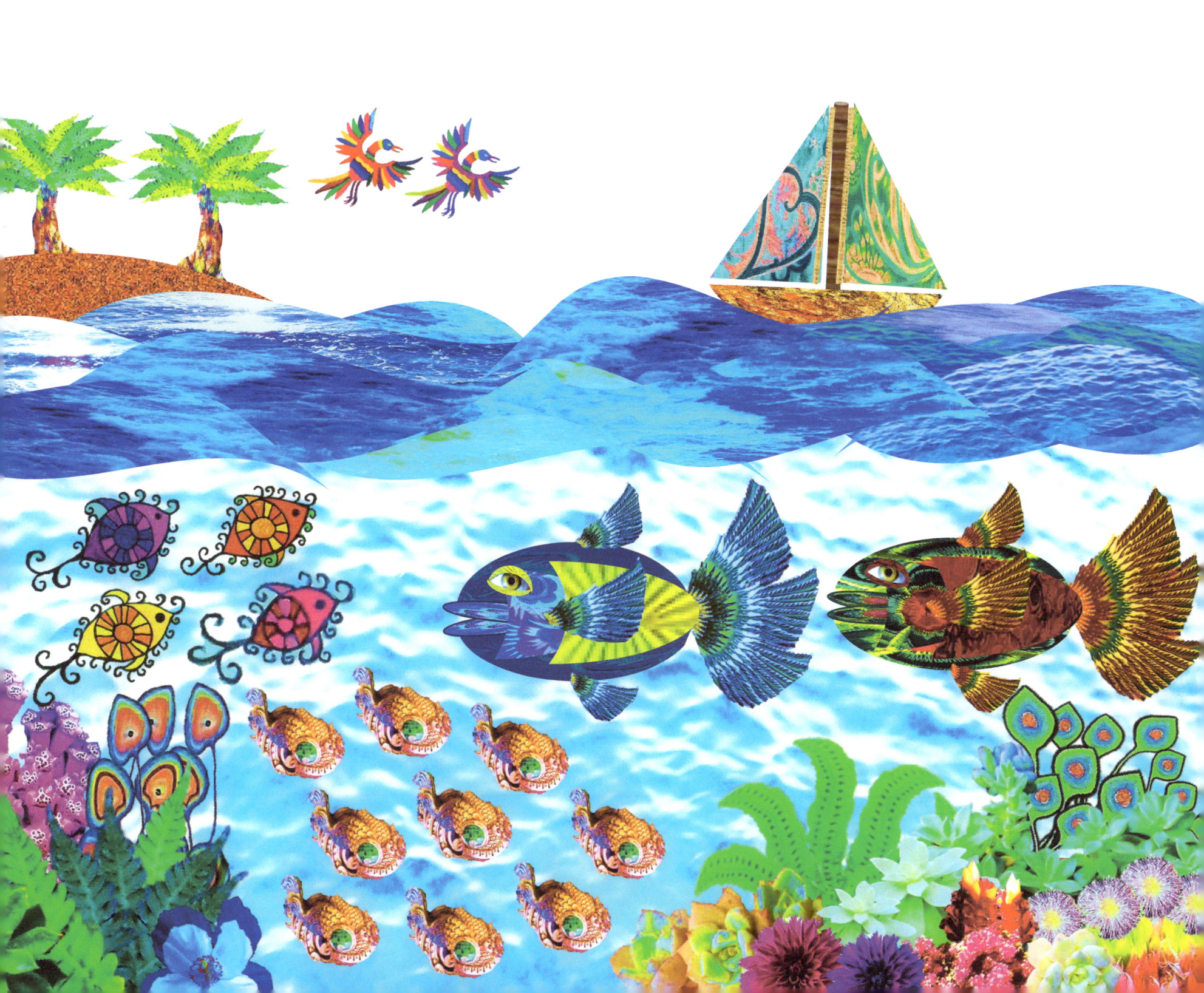

We will pledge our allegiance to unity.

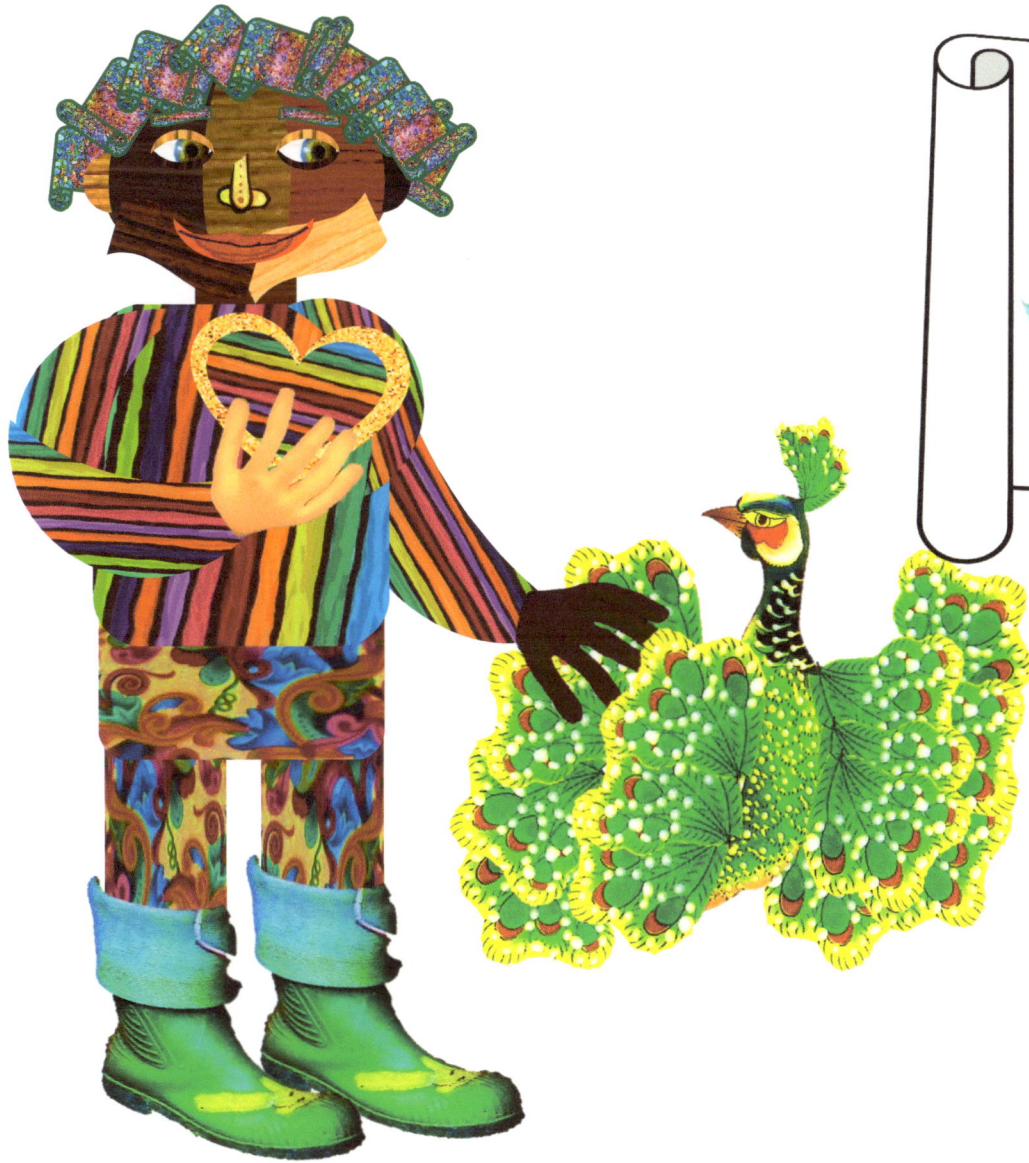

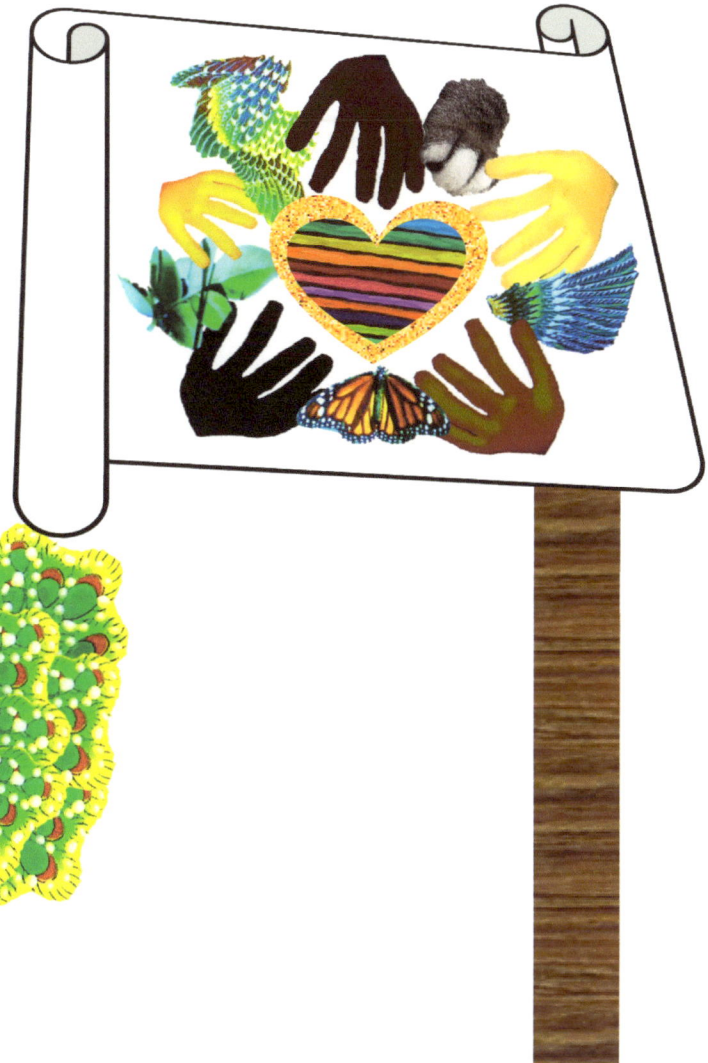

We will remember
with tenderness
the tenderhearted.

You gave...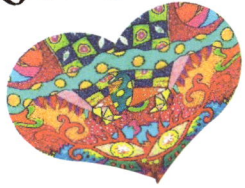

I'm grateful.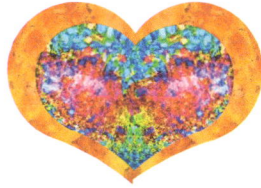

You were...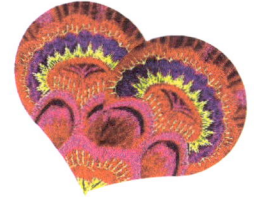

I remember how you...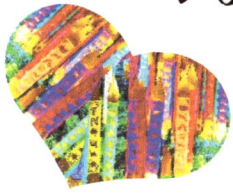

I'm grateful that you...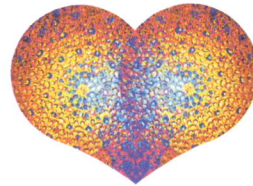

I remember when we...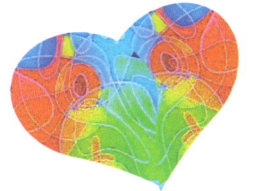

You are always with me.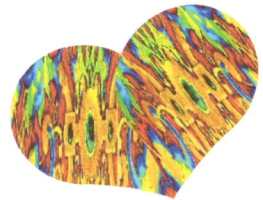

I'm grateful that we...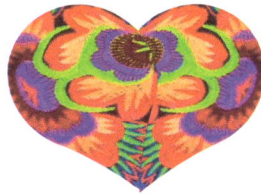

I am always with you.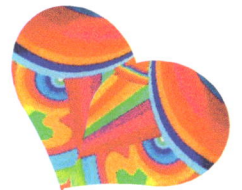

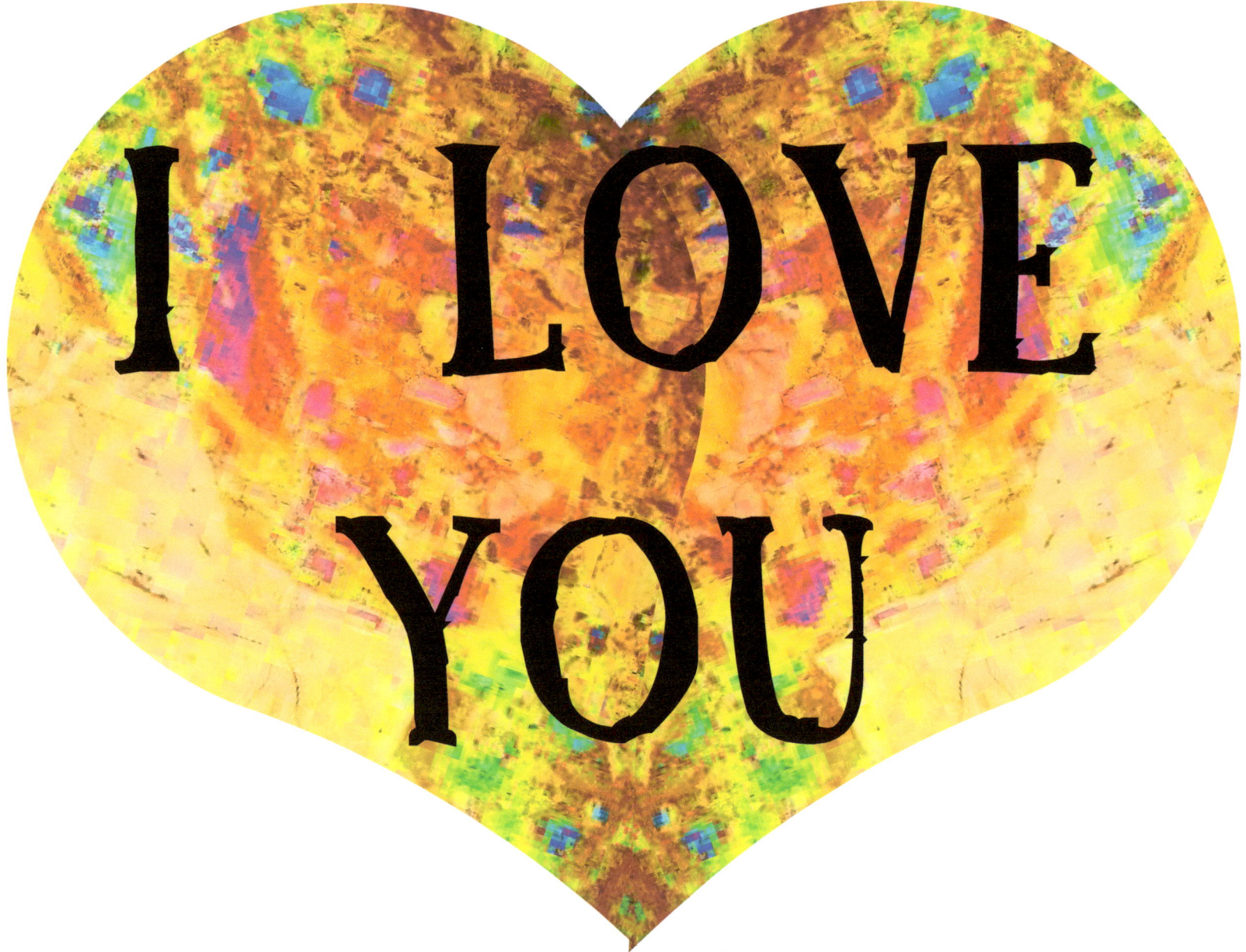

I LOVE YOU

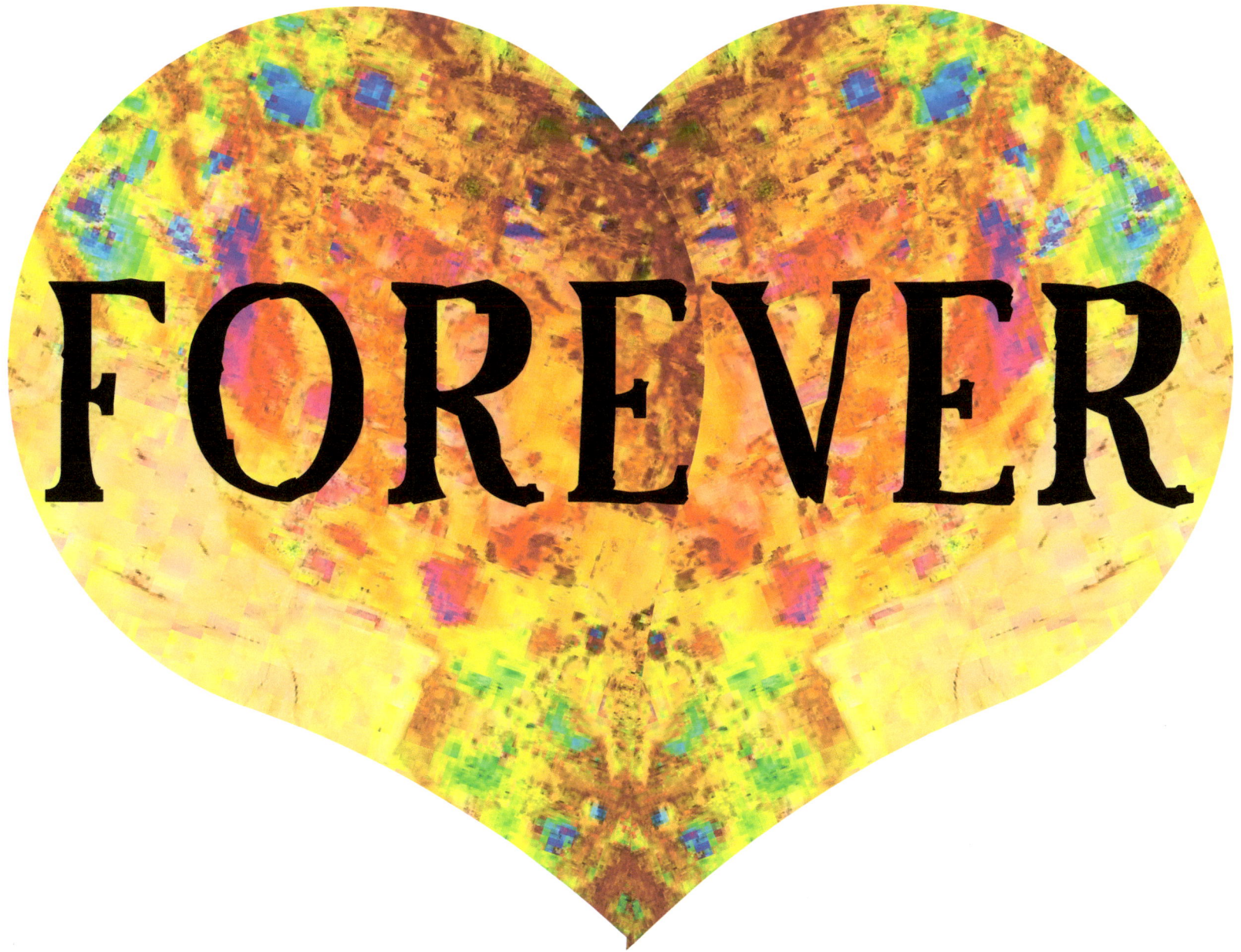

Healing will not be a hope but a certainty
and it will replace stigma
as we reclaim our title of teacher

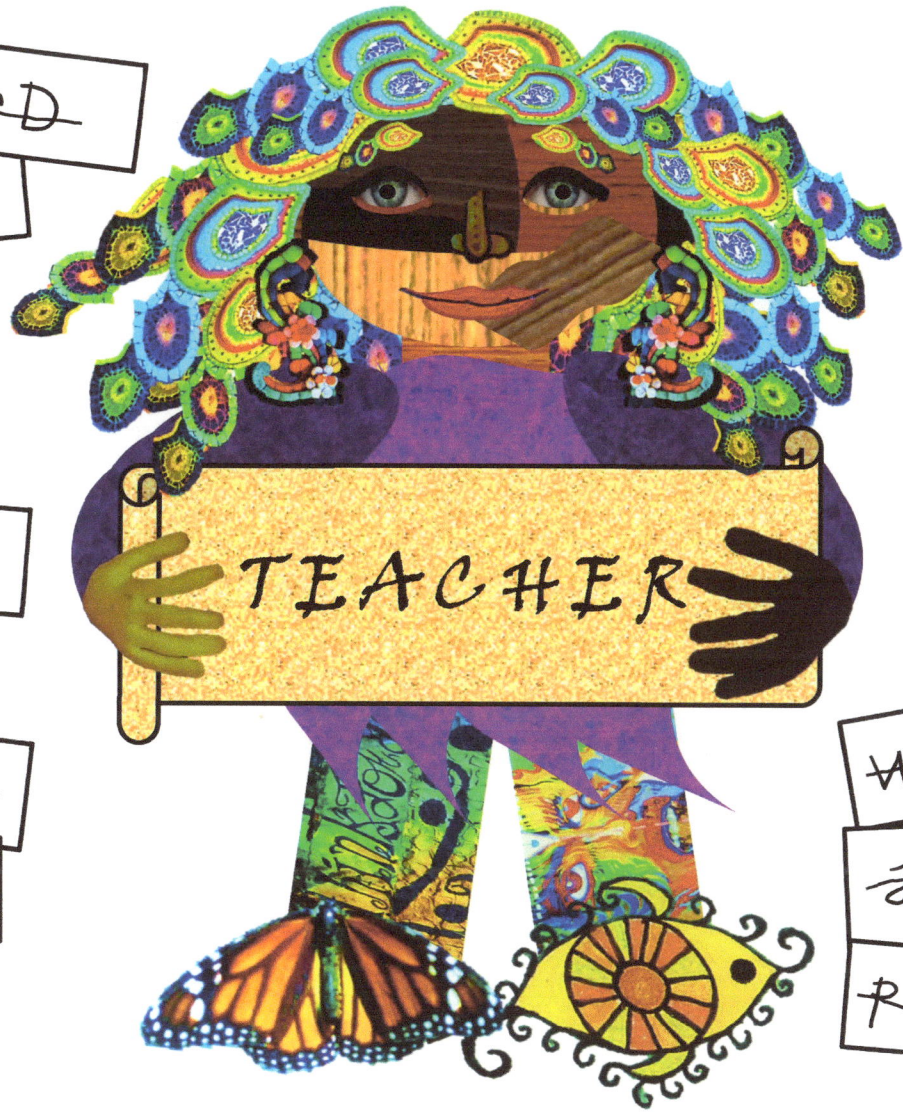

and share with grateful students
what it's like to see through our eyes.

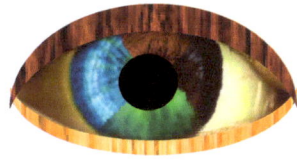

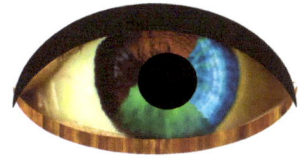

We who have survived on the borders

Welcome!
Food,
homes,
clothing,
and
friendship
for those
who
look,
act,
talk,
and
think like us!
Documents
required.

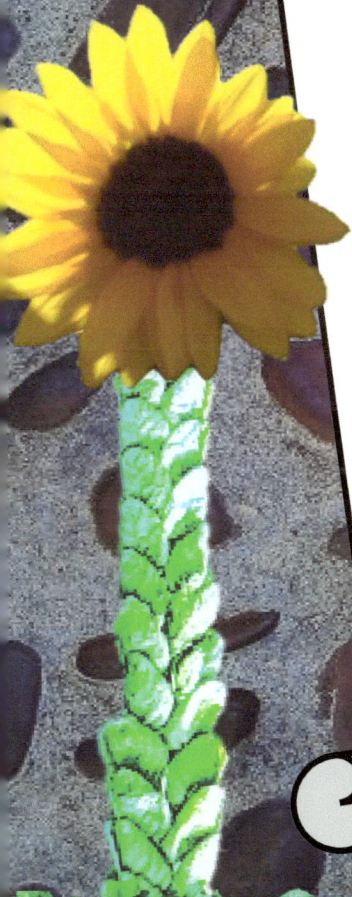

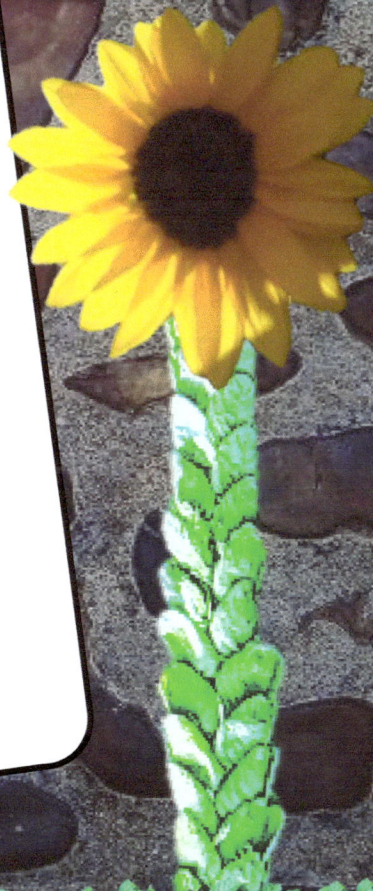

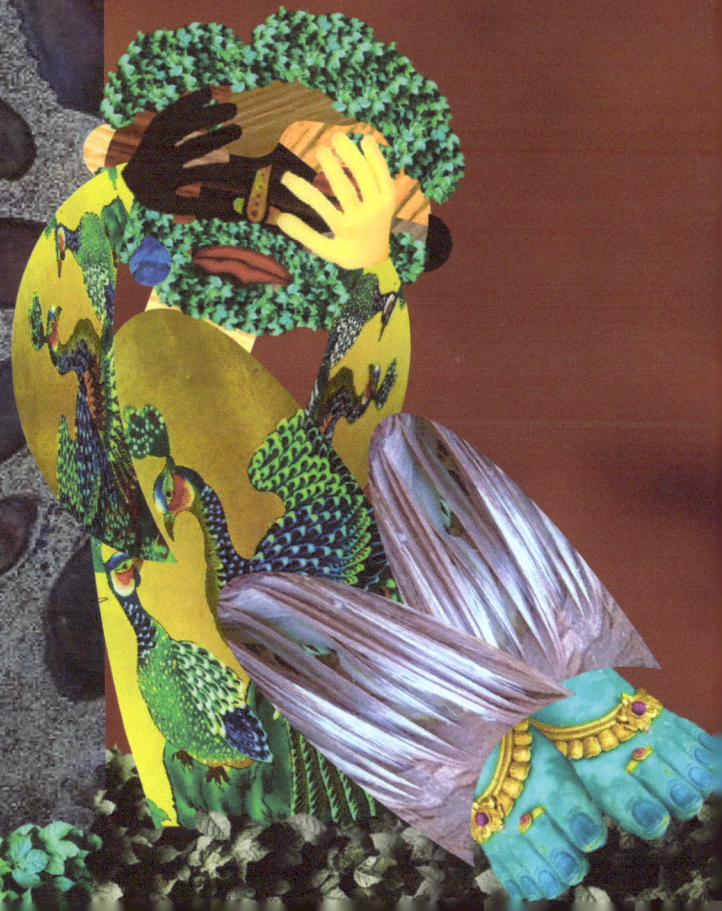

and the precipice of the abyss

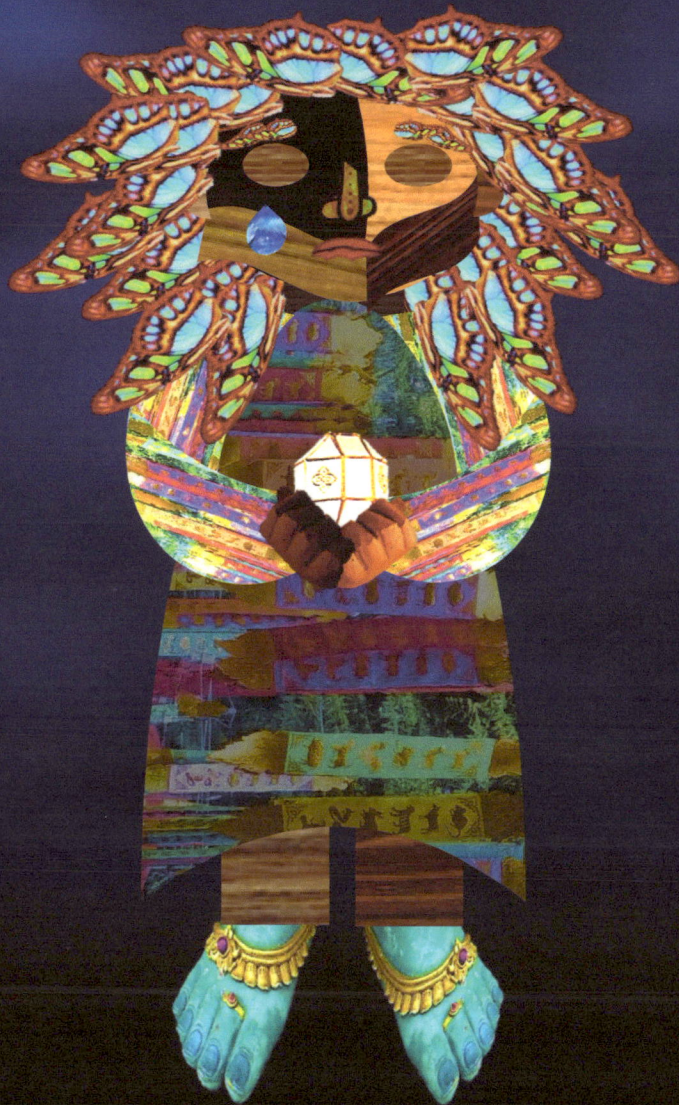

will receive a royal welcome back

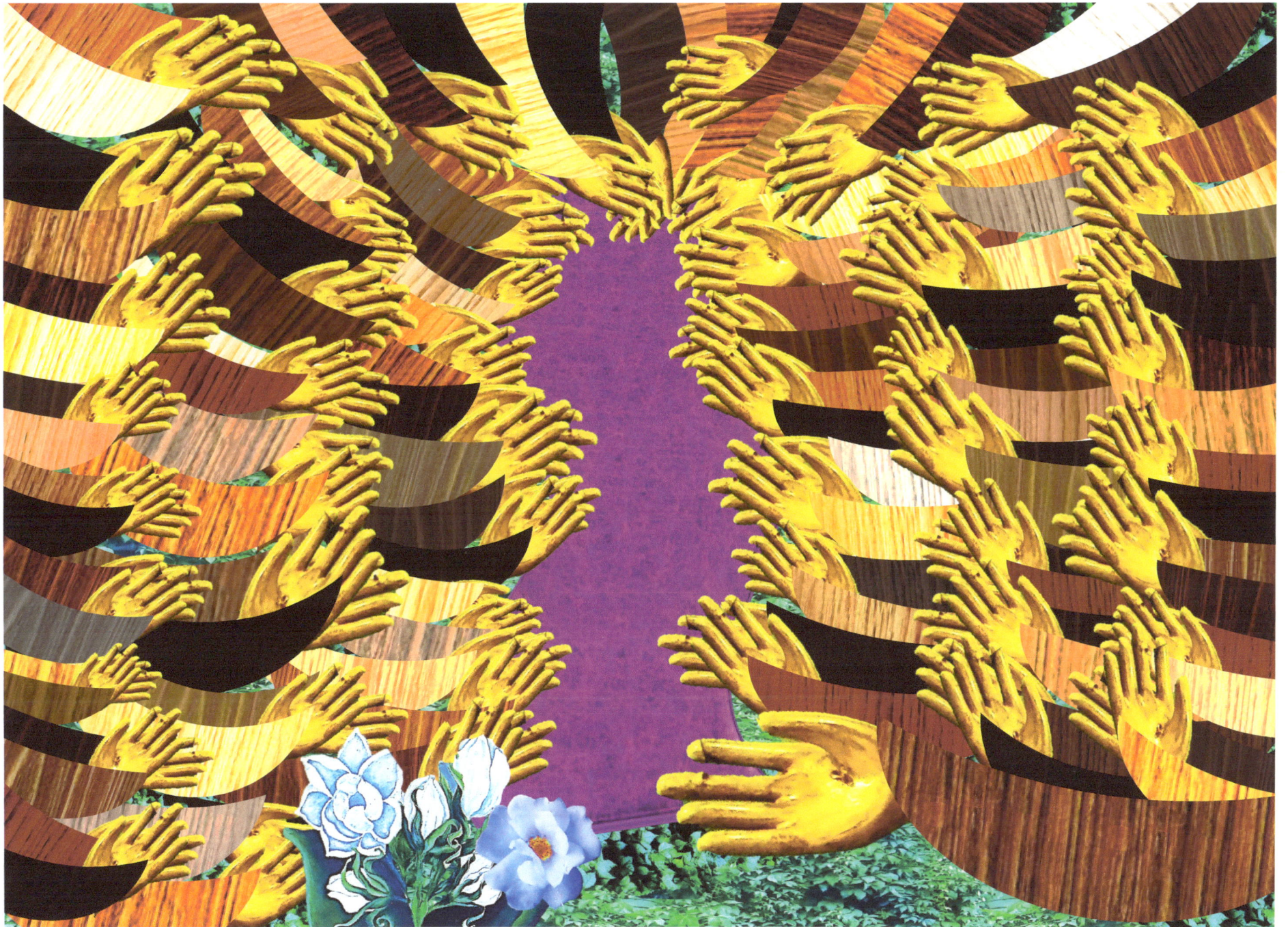

to our royal home:
the union with ALL.

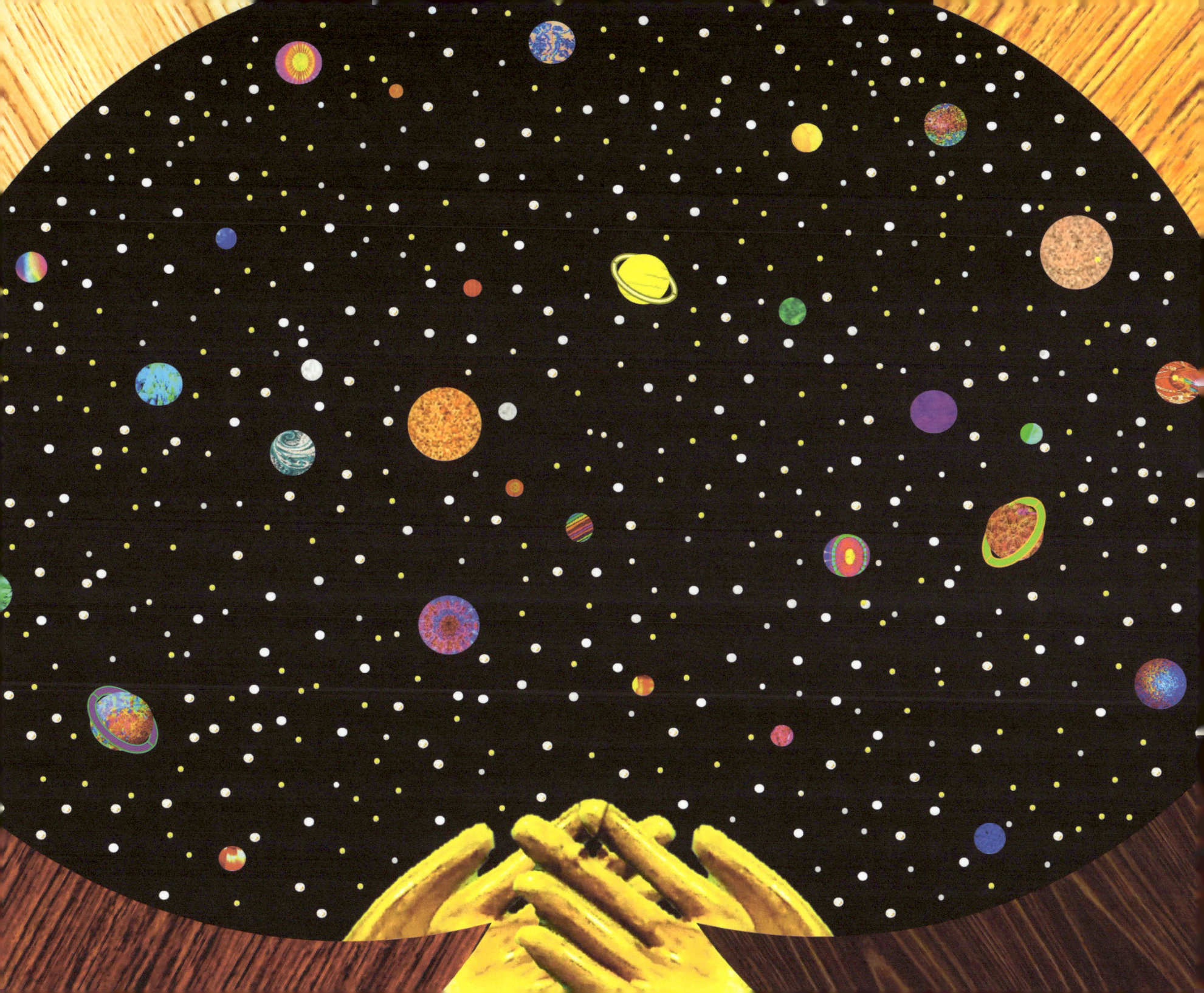

And scars will look back on their ancestors
with the knowledge
that wounds are where they came from
but not where they're headed.

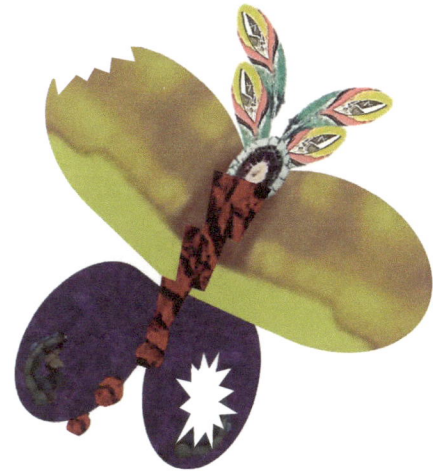

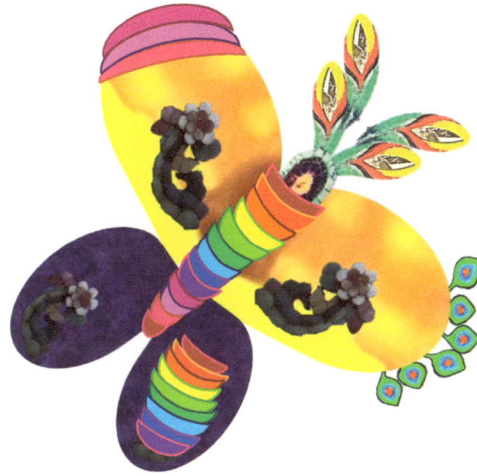

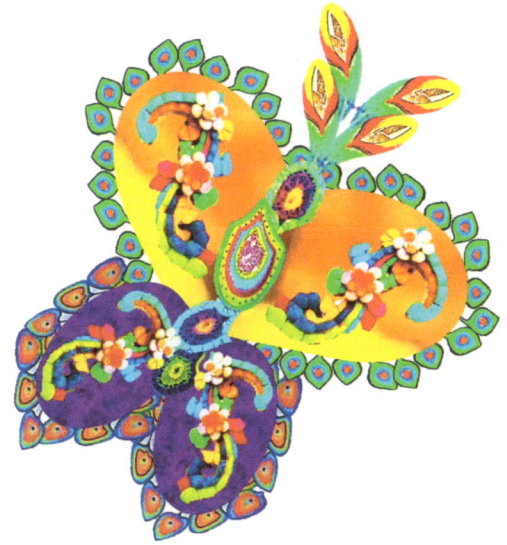

*The new normal.*

The words set me dreaming.
And if these dreams accompany me
from slumber to wakefulness,
I will do with my life what
all freed dragons do with theirs:
I will guide my flight with my flames.

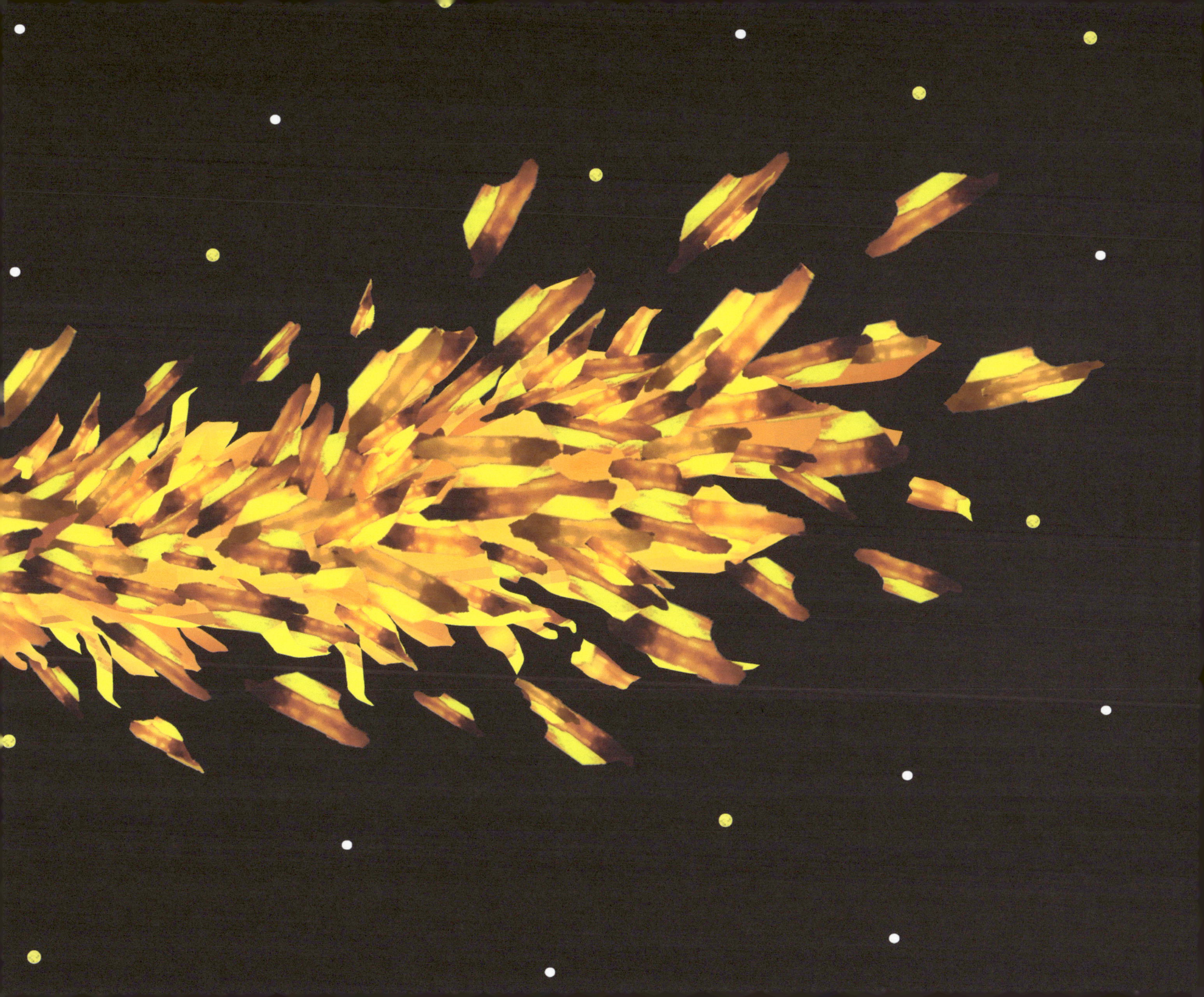

I will be proof that wings can be mended.

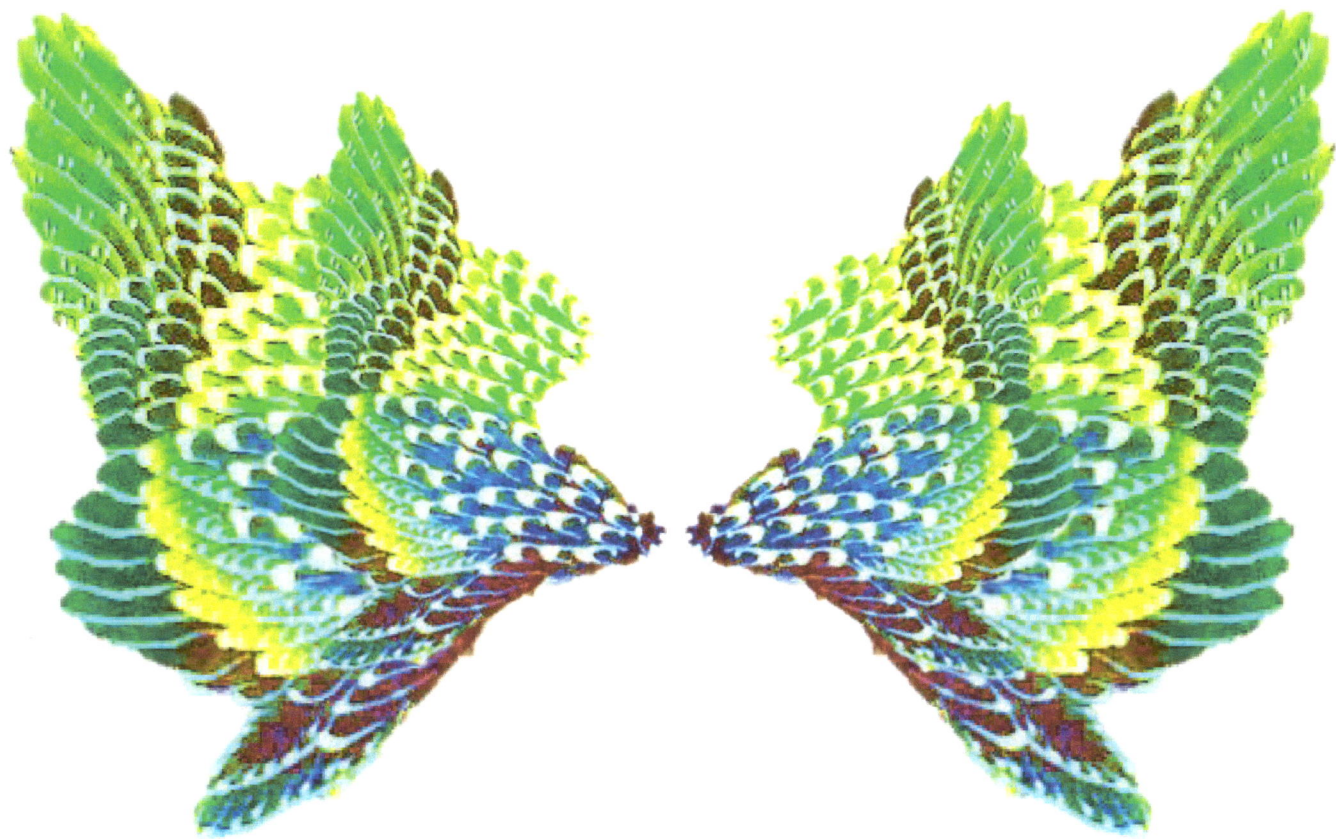

I will reduce to ashes
all the lies decreed laws.

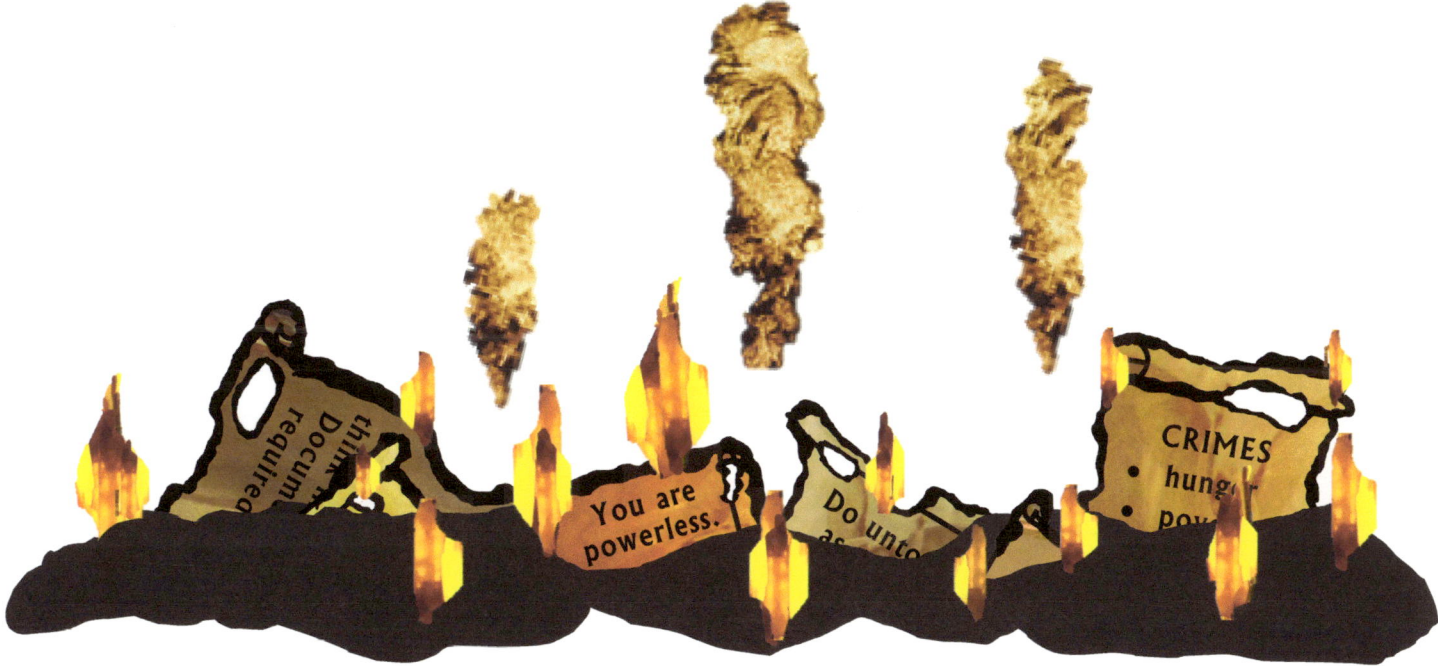

I will be part of the building of something better.

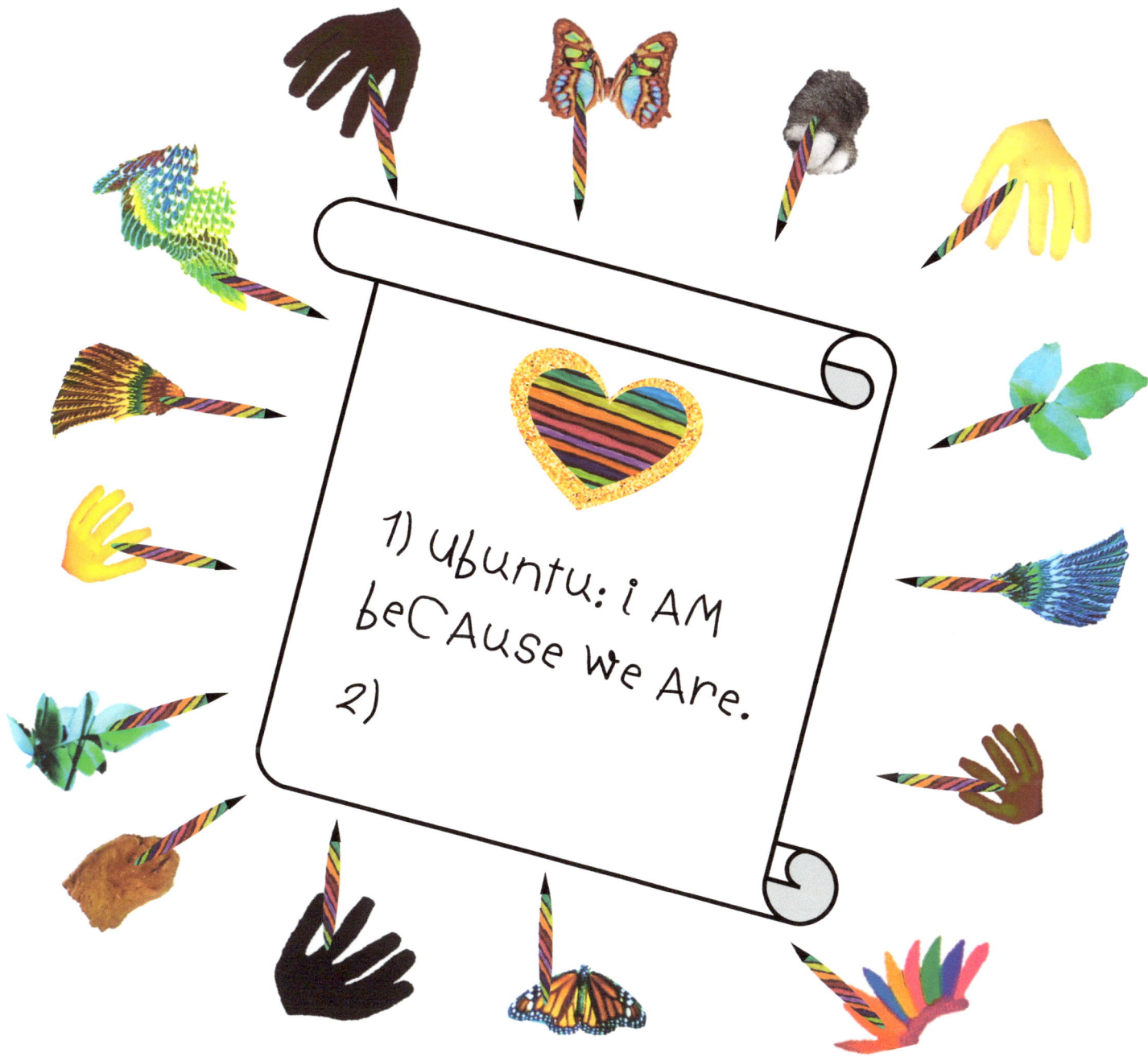

1) ubuntu: i AM beCAuse we Are.

2)

I will soar and roar the word
*PROUD*
at the edge of the night and the cusp of the day
when every heavenly light shines,
so my blessed saviors and former jailers
can see my victory lap.

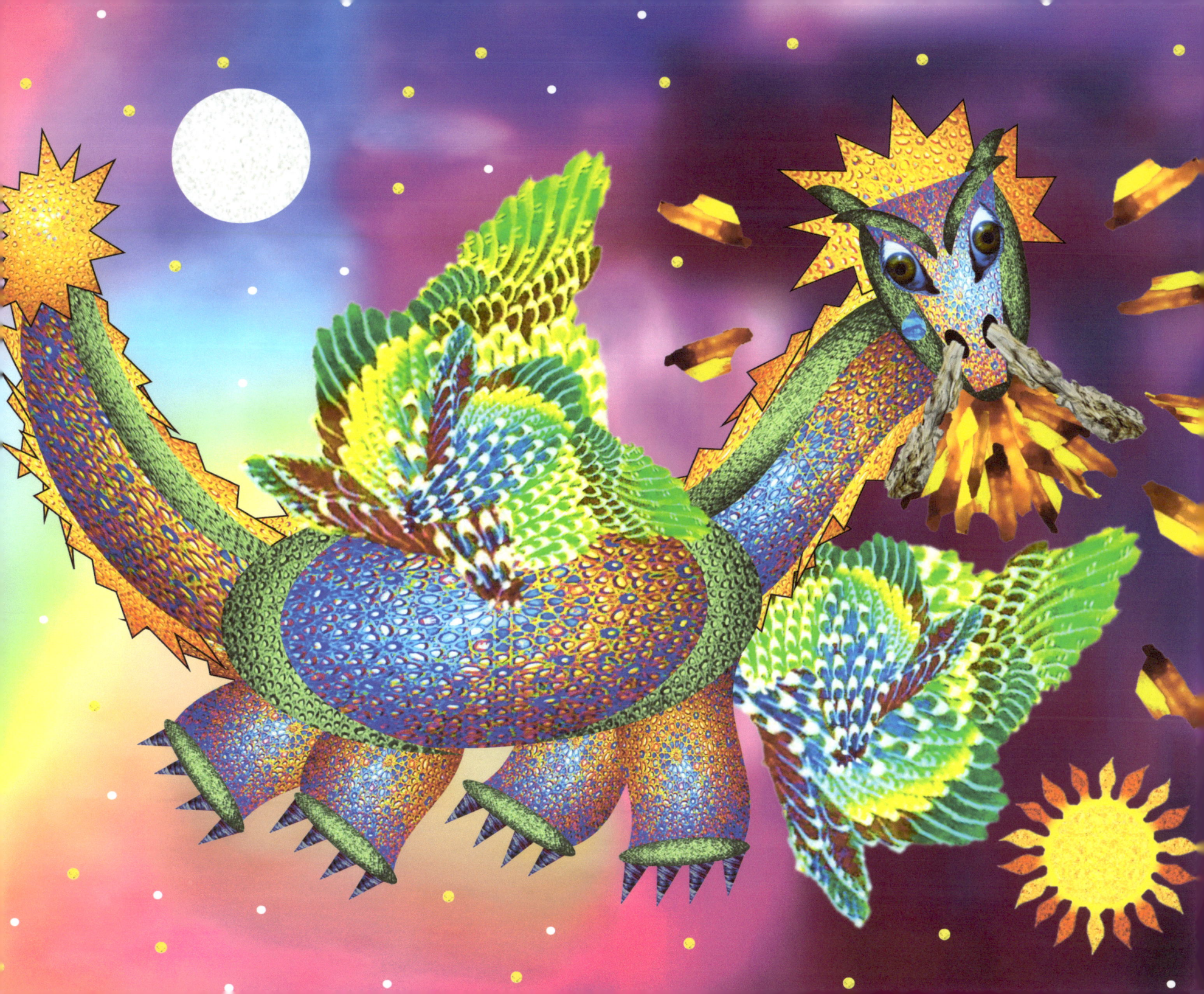

And the clouds will merge with
my smoke-penned letters in the sky,
and the sun, moon, and stars will illumine
what has been spelled,
so the most timid hearts and
the most black-and-blue souls
can read our word writ large:

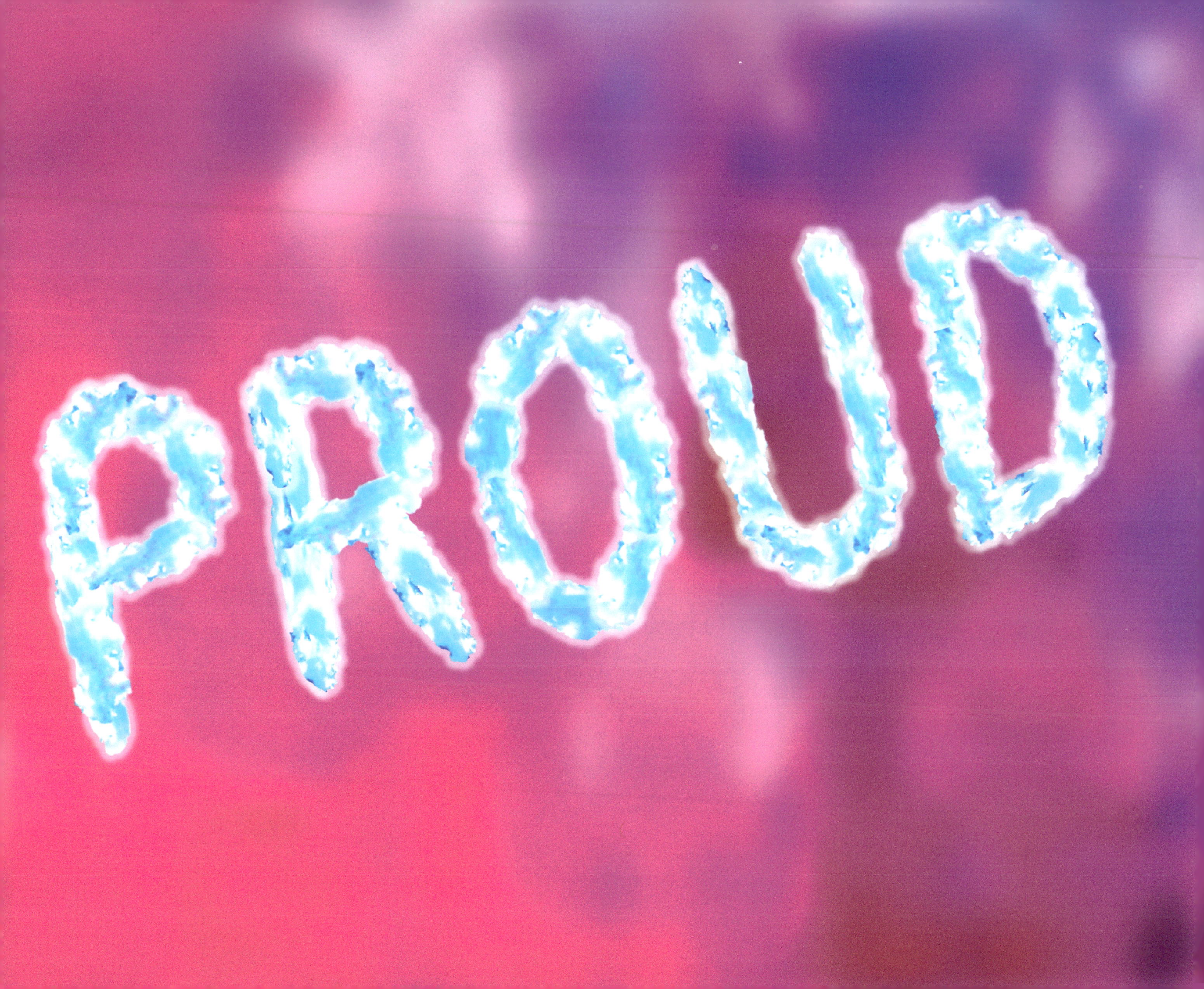
PROUD

A restoration of truth.
A path back to sanity and song.
A rallying cry.
And a reminder
for those who do not believe
they are worthy.

Then I will join my companions in flight
as I sing,

"A radiant life gleams before me,
for I have been reborn."

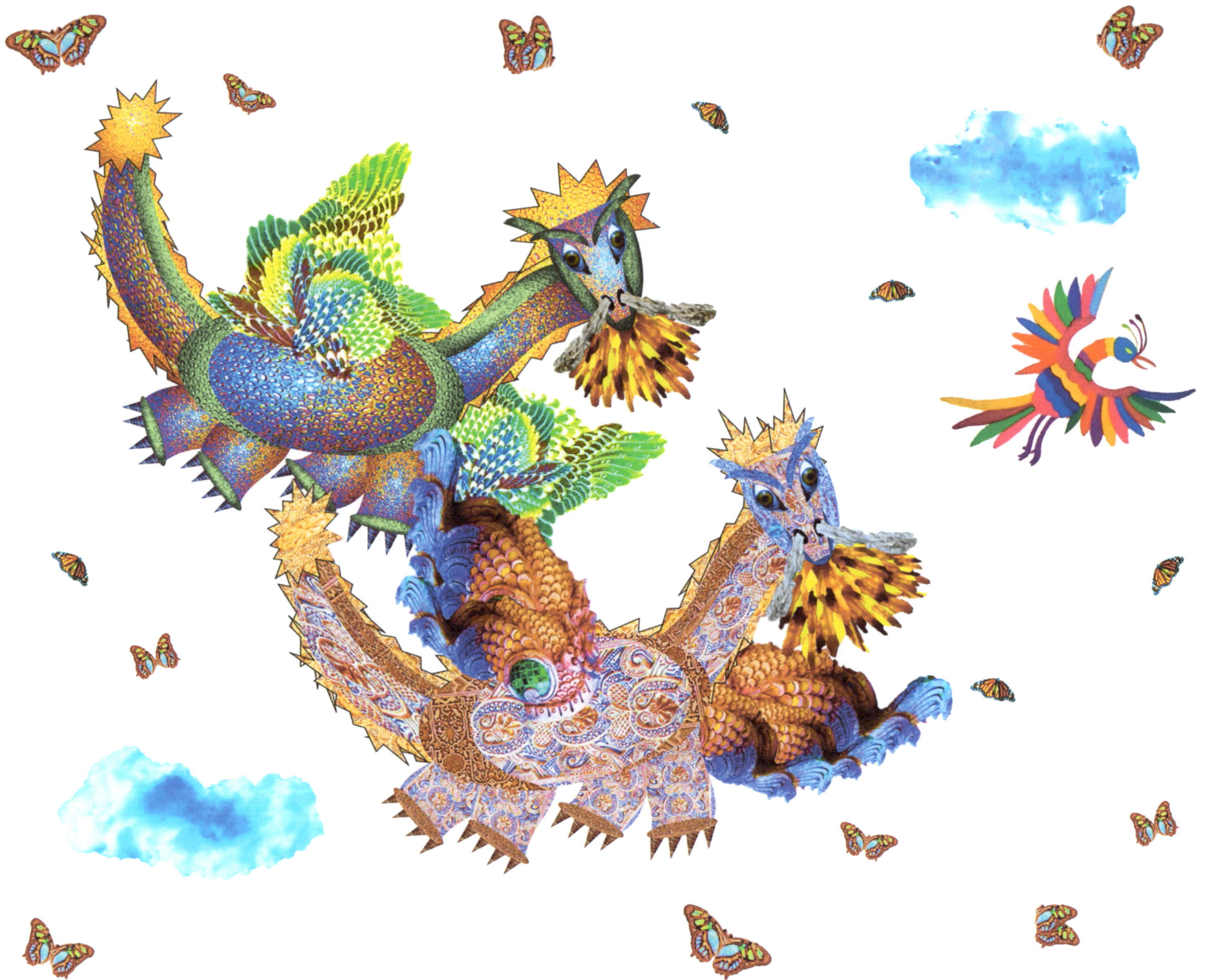

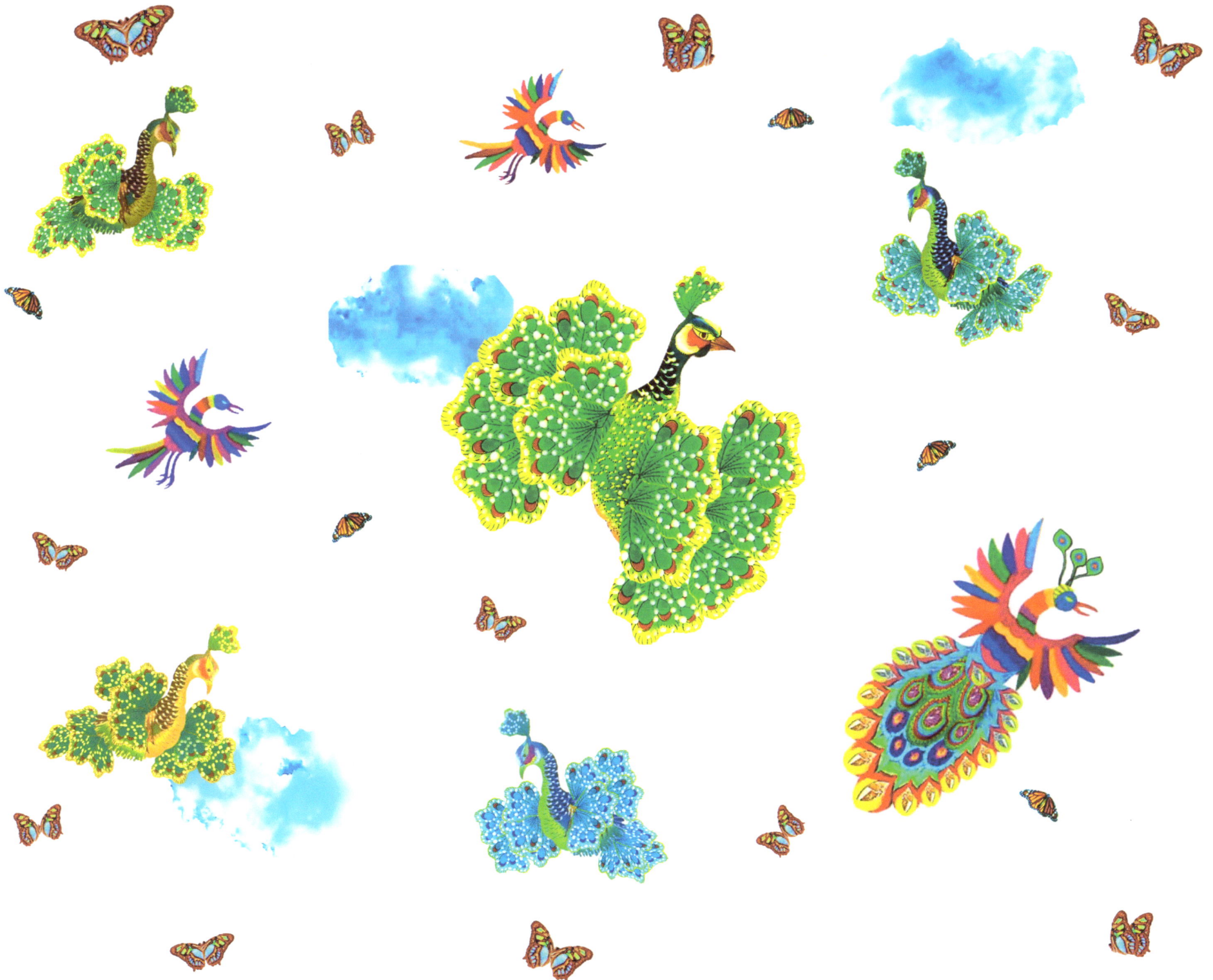

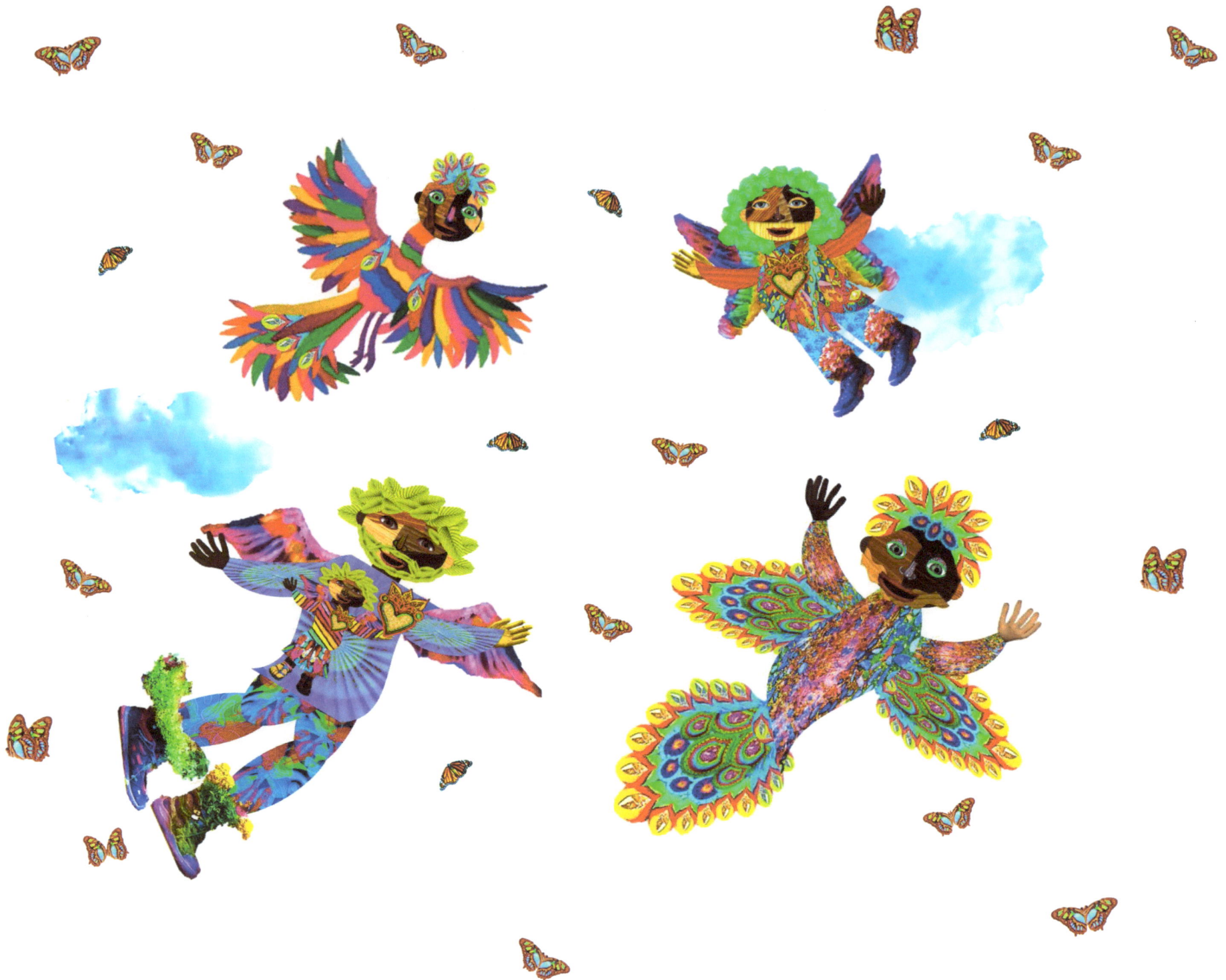

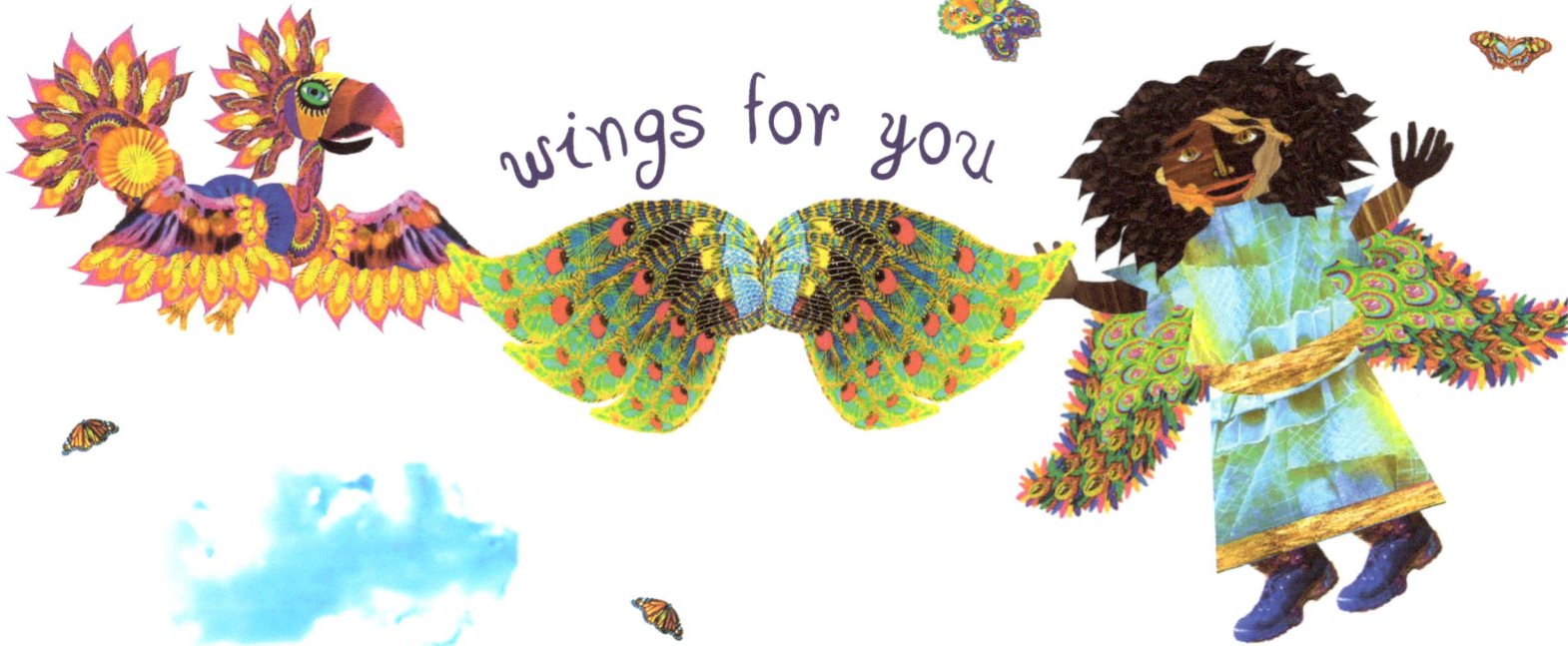

wings for you

it CAn be A revolution...

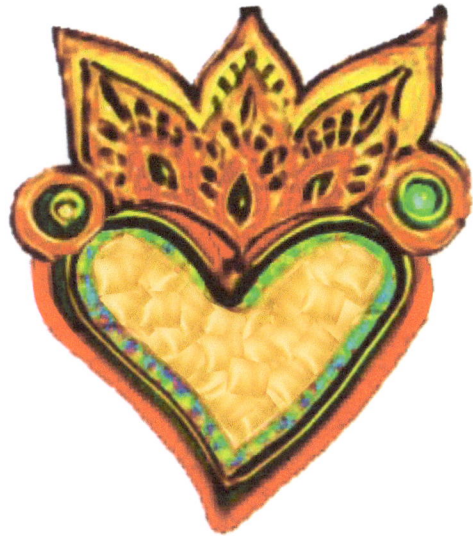